Comparative Physiology of
RENAL EXCRETION

UNIVERSITY REVIEWS IN BIOLOGY

General Editor: J. E. TREHERNE
Advisory Editors: T. WEIS-FOGH
M. J. WELLS   Sir VINCENT WIGGLESWORTH, F.R.S.

ALREADY PUBLISHED

OTHER VOLUMES ARE IN PREPARATION

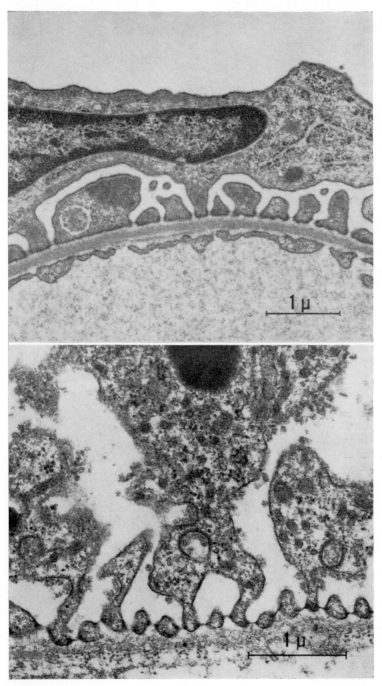

Frontispiece. Upper figure. The region of juxtaposition of podocytes of the visceral epithelium of Bowman's capsule and the capillary endothelium in the rat glomerulus. Lower figure. The region of juxtaposition of epithelial podocytes and haemocoelar spaces in the end sac of the maxillary gland of the brine shrimp. Photomicrographs supplied through the courtesy of Dr. Greta E. Tyson.

Comparative Physiology of
RENAL EXCRETION

J. A. RIEGEL

Lecturer in Zoology,
Westfield College, University of London

OLIVER AND BOYD · EDINBURGH

To
PROFESSOR JAMES ARTHUR RAMSAY, FRS
teacher, critic and friend

OLIVER AND BOYD
Tweeddale Court
14 High Street
Edinburgh EH1 1YL
A Division of Longman Group Limited

ISBN 0 05 002454 x Paperback
    0 05 002455 8 Hardback
First published 1972

Printed in Great Britain by
BELL AND BAIN LTD., GLASGOW

Preface

Comparative Physiology of Renal Excretion is intended to serve both as textbook and review. It is hoped that in addition to its didactic role it will stimulate its readers to enquire further into some of the many areas of ignorance displayed within, either through further reading or their own research. I have tried to portray honestly the state of knowledge of the aspects of renal physiology which have been reviewed, and for most invertebrate renal organs this has been easy, since the number of studies is quite limited. However, for vertebrate renal organs the task has been difficult. Not only are there an enormous number of studies, but many of them present conflicting results. I have attempted to represent fairly all major opinions of those concepts which are in conflict, but doubtless this will not be seen to be the case by the various advocates!

In the preparation of the book, I have received help from many persons. Chief amongst these is my wife, who helped at all stages. Professor J. E. Webb, Dr. J. M. Skelding and Miss June Mason reviewed the entire manuscript and Professor Klaus Thurau reviewed Chapter 6. Dr. Greta Tyson very kindly supplied the frontispiece and original illustrations for Fig. 35A–D. Dr. John Skelding furnished original drawings for Fig. 39 and permitted me to quote from his unpublished studies. Miss P. A. Keefe (Mrs. Farquharson) and Mr. M. R. Phillips permitted me to quote from their unpublished studies. Mr. John Rodford redrew certain of the figures. Dr. John Treherne, the series editor, helped me with many of the technical details of manuscript preparation. To all of the foregoing persons, I extend my gratitude, and, of course, I absolve them of blame for any defects which remain. To the authors and publishers who permitted me to use illustrations from their publications, I extend my thanks. The details are listed on pages *ix* to *xi*. Finally, it was Dr. John Treherne who first suggested that I write this book. Now that the task is completed, I forgive him.

J. A. RIEGEL

Westfield College
October, 1971

Contents

Acknowledgements

The writer gratefully acknowledges the authors and publishers who have given permission to use the illustrations whose details are listed below.

In this book		Source	Author(s)	Publisher	In the source	
Fig. No.	Ref. No.				Vol. and Page	Fig. No.
1	62	Q. Jl. Microsc. Sci.	Goodrich	Company of Biologists	88:124, 125	5 7
2	77	Fish Physiology	Hickman, Trump	Academic Press, Inc.	1:213	46
3A	190	Am. J. Physiol.	Schmidt-Nielsen, O'Dell	American Physiological Society	200:1121	2
3B	65	Am. J. Med.	Gottschalk	Rueben H. Donnelly Corpn.	36:673	3
4A 7	171	Proc. Roy. Soc. Lond., B	Richards	Royal Society of London	126:419, 415	15A 13
4B	60	Am. J. Med.	Giebisch Windhager	Reuben H. Donnelly Corpn.	36:647 644, 646 656	3 1, 2 9
10, 11 13						
8	225	Acta Soc. med. Upsal.	Wallenius	Medical Society, Uppsala	59:21, 76	3, 20
12	202	Am. J. Physiol.	Spitzer, Windhager	American Physiological Society	218:1189	1
14	84	J. clin. Invest.	Jaenike, Berliner	American Society for Clinical Investigations	39:485	5

Acknowledgements *cont.*

In this book			Author(s)	Publisher	In the source	
Fig. No.	Ref. No.	Source			Vol. and Page	Fig. No.
15 left	150	*J. cell. comp. Physiol.*	Pitts	Wistar Institute	11:105	3
15 right	52	*J. gen. Physiol.*	Forster, Hong	Rockefeller Univ. Press	45:815	2
16A, B	193	*Am. J. Physiol.*	Silverman, Aganon, Chinard	American Physiological Society	218:736	1, 2
16C					738	4
19	21	*Tissue and Cell*	Berridge, Oschman	Longman Group, Ltd.	1:247–272	various
20	161	*J. exp. Biol.*	Ramsay	Company of Biologists	29:116	3
21	165	*J. exp. Biol.*	Ramsay	Company of Biologists	32:207	2
22	167	*J. exp. Biol.*	Ramsay	Company of Biologists	35:880	1
23	114	*J. exp. Biol.*	Maddrell	Company of Biologists	51:85	12
24					90	14
25	83	*Am. J. Physiol.*	Irvine	American Physiological Society	217:1524	6
26	17	*J. exp. Biol.*	Berridge	Company of Biologists	50:19	5
27	14	*J. insect Physiol.*	Berridge	Pergamon Press	12:1535	11
28	15	*Insects and Physiology*	Berridge	Oliver and Boyd	page 334	2
29A	71	*J. Morph.*	Gupta, Berridge	Wistar Institute	120:45	plate 1
29B, C	69	*Phil. Trans. Roy. Soc. Lond.*, B	Grimstone, Mullinger, Ramsay	Royal Society of London	253:346	2, 1
30	144	*J. exp. Biol.*	Phillips	Company of Biologists	41:25	4B
31	168	*Phil. Trans. Roy. Soc. Lond.*, B	Ramsay	Royal Society of London	248:303	14B
32	69	*Phil. Trans. Roy. Soc. Lond.*, B	Grimstone, Mullinger, Ramsay	Royal Society of London	253:37	443

x

33	223	Am. J. Physiol.	Wall, Oschman	American Physiological Society	218:1212	6
35A-D	214	Z. Zellforsch. (Histochemie)	Tyson	Springer-Verlag	93:160	13A-D
36	32	Biol. Bull., Woods Hole	Burger	Marine Biological Assoc., Woods Hole	113:209 211	1 3
37	177	J. exp. Biol.	Riegel	Company of Biologists	48:592	2
38	153	Biol. Rev.	Potts	Cambridge Univ. Press	42:3, 4 6, 7	1, 2 3A, 4
40	126	J. exp. Biol.	Martin, Stewart, Harrison	Company of Biologists	42:107	7
41, 42	75	J. exp. Biol.	Harrison, Martin	Company of Biologists	42:85, 89 90	10, 16 17
43	152	Comp. Biochem. Physiol.	Potts	Pergamon Press	14:348	4
44	103	J. exp. Biol.	Little	Company of Biologists	43:48	7B
45A, B	68	Zool. Beitr.	Graszinski	Duncker and Humblot	8:200 268	1 12
46, 47A 47B	23	Z. vergl. Physiol.	Boroffka	Springer-Verlag	51:35, 36 37	7, 8 9
48	24	Z. vergl. Physiol.	Boroffka, Altner, Haupt	Springer-Verlag	66:423, 431	1 7
50A, B	94	Sekretion und Exkretion	Kümmel	Springer-Verlag	pp. 207 221	2A 10A
51	192	J. Protozool.	Schneider	Society of Protozoologists	7:76	1
52A	37	J. gen. Physiol.	Curran	Rockefeller Univ. Press	43:1146	5
52B	21	Tissue and Cell	Berridge, Oschman	Longman Group, Ltd.	1:265	18
53	53	J. Physiol.	Frederiksen, Leyssac	The Physiological Society	201:221	11
54A	180	Comp. Biochem. Physiol.	Riegel	Pergamon Press	36:405	1

Part 1: An Introduction to Renal Physiology

Chapter 1

Excretion is a somewhat ambiguous term, meaning, literally, 'a sorting out.' A great variety of tissues and organs excrete, including kidneys. The terms 'kidney' and 'renal organ' are fairly unambiguous in their usage as general morphological descriptions of organs which produce urine. Therefore, where possible, the specific or general name (e.g., antennal gland, protonephridium) of kidneys will be used, but where these terms are not well known (e.g., organ of Bojanus in the lamellibranch molluscs), the term kidney or renal organ will be used.

This review will concentrate on kidneys whose function has been investigated experimentally. Invertebrate renal physiology has consisted of a search for functions analogous to those known or thought to occur in vertebrate renal organs. In order to understand invertebrate physiology, it is thus first necessary to have an elementary knowledge of vertebrate renal physiology.

The kinds of kidneys

The primitive kidneys of the Eumetazoa are derived from one or both of two tubes which develop during embryogeny[62]. The first of these tubes develops centripetally ('out to in') and is given the name nephridium. The second tube develops centrifugally ('in to out') and is called a coelomoduct. In many cases, the renal organ represents a combination of nephridium and coelomoduct, in which case it is called a nephromixium. It must be emphasized that the foregoing are morphological terms and relate to the embryological origin of the kidneys.

Nephridia

Nephridia, which function primitively as true kidneys, are of two basic types. Protonephridia (Fig. 1A) are considered to be unicellular and closed at their terminal ends; they bear one or more tufts of cilia (flame cell) or a single flagellum (solenocyte). The cilia and flagella beat or undulate in the extracellular space, giving a 'flickering' appearance when viewed under a microscope, hence the name, flame cell.

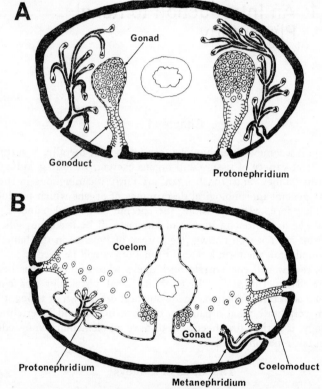

FIG. 1.   Origin of the body cavity (coelom) in animals, and the relationship of nephridia and coelomoducts to the body cavity. A. Coelomate animal (flatworm). Protonephridia (flame cells) are present, as are coelomoducts which convey sex cells from the gonad to the outside of the body. B. Coelomate animal (annelid). The gonadal cavity has expanded to become the coelom. The protonephridia (solenocytes, left of figure) and metanephridia have penetrated the coelomic space. Modified from Goodrich.[62]

The metanephridium (Fig. 1B) represents a tube which opens into the coelomic space by a ciliated funnel, the nephridiostome.

Coelomoducts

Coelomoducts are outgrowths from the coelom which serve primitively to carry gonadal products.[62] The concept of the coelomoduct fits readily into the 'gonocoel' theory of the origin of the coelom, propounded first by Hatscheck and elaborated by Goodrich and others. According to this theory, the coelom arose by an expansion of the gonadal cavity. Thus the coelomoduct represents a persistant gonadal duct. The coelomoduct gave rise to the renal organs of a wide variety of coelomate animals, including vertebrates (Fig. 2). The metanephridium looks superficially like a coelomoduct because it opens to the coelom. However, this occurs secondarily by the penetration of the end of the metanephridium into the coelomic space.

The importance of the foregoing discussion lies primarily in the insight it gives into the seemingly highly variable morphology of renal organs. Amongst the animals to be discussed, vertebrates, arthropods and molluscs possess coelomoduct-derived kidneys. With the exception of the protozoans, the remainder possess nephridial kidneys. Very frequently the kidneys of arthropods and molluscs are called nephridia, but patently they are not. Nephridium is a morphological term and its use should be confined to morphological descriptions. When a functional term is to be used, 'renal organ', 'kidney' or even 'excretory organ' should be used.

The Malpighian tubules of arthropods do not fit into the Goodrich scheme. They appear to be developed independently of either nephridia or coelomoducts. In fact, in some arthropods, such as primitive insects (e.g. the spring-tails or *Collembola*) myriapods and arachnids, the Malpighian tubules occur in addition to well-developed coelomoduct-derived renal organs.

The origin and elaboration of vertebrate nephrons

The development of the vertebrate kidney has been reviewed adequately by Goodrich.[63] During a brief period in the embryogeny of the vertebrate nephron, there is a stage which resembles the coelomoduct. The embryonic nephron consists of a winding tubule leading to a duct (pronephric duct), which leads to the outside of the embryo. The winding tubule opens to the coelomic space by a ciliated funnel.

Amongst the vertebrate classes, the nephrons exhibit a high degree of variability with respect to the presence or absence of segments which are histologically and perhaps physiologically distinct. Nowhere is this variability more apparent than in the fishes. Most fortunately, the review recently published by Hickman and Trump[77] is an admirable synthesis of an immense amount of data which hitherto was scattered widely in the literature. Here we shall briefly summarize one aspect of this review, namely, the synthesis of possible homologies and evolutionary trends in vertebrate nephrons. The reader is urged to read the full review.

Evolutionary trends in the vertebrate nephron

The scheme of Hickman and Trump is based primarily upon the increasing osmoregulatory efficiency of vertebrate nephrons (Fig. 2). Briefly, the evolution of the nephron is considered to have occurred along three main lines. The initial stage of development may have existed in a hypothetical 'protovertebrate' (Fig. 2a), where filtration occurred out of a blood vessel into the adjacent coelom. The coelom communicated with the exterior of the animal by a simple excretory pore. A second stage of development of the vertebrate nephron (also hypothetical) may have consisted of a structure which was incompletely separated from the coelom (Fig. 2b). This condition approaches the coelomoduct stage envisaged by Goodrich. The primitive nephron was adjacent to a specialized circulatory component. Fluid was filtered into the nephron which communicated both with the coelom, by a nephrostome, and with the exterior of the body. The third stage (Fig. 2c) represents the condition found in the mesonephrons of modern hagfish (myxinoid cyclostomes). Here the nephron exists as a discrete unit with a glomerulus, neck segment and tubule; the tubule is thought to be homologous with the proximal tubule of higher vertebrates. The glomerulus is a specialized structure in which blood vessels and the head of the renal tubule are intimately associated. The next stage in the evolutionary sequence of the vertebrate nephron may be the basic plan of the first vertebrates to enter freshwater; it is represented here by the nephron of the anadromous lamprey (Fig. 2d). Here the collecting tubule was added, which, presumably, was essential for the formation of dilute urine. The next two stages (Figs. 2f, g) represent the addition of segments to the nephron, presumably to increase the osmoregulatory efficiency in freshwater animals. These two stages may have been the beginnings of a line of evolution which continued with semiterrestrial animals (amphibians, Fig. 2k) and culminated with mammals (Fig. 2l). Elaboration of the nephron in groups more highly evolved than amphibians probably proceeded by differential growth of pre-existing nephron segments (e.g. the intermediate segment developed into the loop of Henle) and by specializations of the arrangements of the nephrons

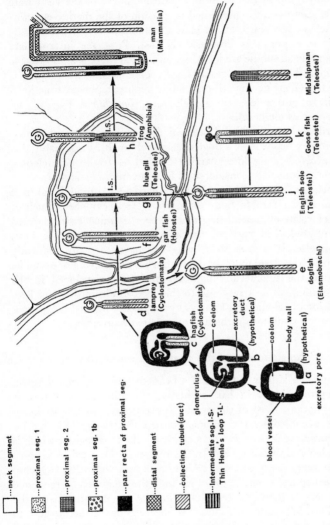

Fig. 2. Evolutionary development of the vertebrate nephron. The nephron may have developed from a primitive state in which filtration occurred from blood vessels in the body wall directly into the coelom. The coelom was drained by a simple excretory pore (a). This stage approximates to the coelomoduct. The next series of stages (b–d) saw the development of a specialized filtration apparatus, the glomerulus, and its association with a specialized excretory duct. Further evolutionary development may have occurred along three lines: development of the complex elasmobranch nephron (e); development of the complex nephron of freshwater fishes which led to nephrons of semiterrestrial (amphibian) and terrestrial animals (f–i); regression of the nephron after reinvasion of the sea (j–l). Probable homologies of the nephron parts are keyed in the homology code. Modified from Hickman and Trump.[77]

G ...glomerulus

...neck segment

...proximal seg. 1

...proximal seg. 2

...proximal seg. 1b

...pars recta of proximal seg.

...distal segment

...collecting tubule (duct)

...intermediate seg. I.S.-
Thin Henle's loop T.-L.

blood vessel

a (hypothetical)
body wall
coelom
excretory pore

b (hypothetical)
excretory duct
coelom
glomerulus

c hagfish (Cyclostomata)

d lamprey (Cyclostomata)

e dogfish (Elasmobranchi)

f gar fish (Holostei)

g blue gill (Teleostei)   I.S.

h frog (Amphibia)   I.S.

i man (Mammalia)

j English sole (Teleostei)

k Goose fish (Teleostei)

l Midshipman (Teleostei)

within the kidney. Thus the complex arrangement into medullary and cortical parts of the kidneys of mammals and some birds may be classified as an arrangement specialization.

A second trend in the evolutionary development of the vertebrate nephron is seen upon the presumed reinvasion of the marine environment by teleost fish (Figs. 2h, j). Here the complex form of the freshwater teleost nephron is progressively lost. First the intermediate segment and distal tubule are lost (Fig. 2h). Then there is a progressive diminution of the number of glomeruli. In some marine teleosts such as the goose fish (*Lophius*, Fig. 2i) only a few nephrons possess functional glomeruli. In others (e.g. the midshipman, *Porichthys*, Fig. 2j), no nephrons possess glomeruli.

A third evolutionary trend seen in fish nephrons is represented by the complex nephron of a dogfish (elasmobranch). Presumably this nephron evolved along lines parallel to that of freshwater teleosts, because both groups are considered to have a common ancestor.

The scheme illustrated in Fig. 2 is extremely useful because it synthesizes a considerable body of morphological evidence, much of which is of relatively recent origin. However, it must be recognised that the physiological basis of the scheme is fragmentary at best. If nothing else, it is true that living organisms are pre-eminently opportunistic: they tend to 'make do' with what they have. For example, even though the aglomerular nephron may have developed in the marine environment as a response to the need to diminish water loss, the possession of aglomerular kidneys by freshwater pipefishes (syngnathids) does not seem to put them at an undue disadvantage.

The structure of the mammalian kidney

The mammalian kidney is typically a bean-shaped or lobulated organ. By cutting the kidney in half sagittally, the following structure is revealed (Fig. 3a). Most of the greater (outer) curvature of the 'bean' or lobe is occupied by the compacted nephric tissue. The interior (medial) curvature is occupied by a chamber, the renal pelvis, which is the expanded end of the ureter. In the region of the renal pelvis may be seen the renal artery and vein which break up into smaller branches within the nephric tissue. Projecting into the chamber of the renal pelvis are one or more pointed elongations of the nephric tissue, the renal papillae. When the half kidney is observed under the medium to high power of a stereoscopic (dissecting) microscope still more detail is revealed. The nephric tissue is divided into two discrete zones, an outer or cortical zone and an inner or medullary zone. The cortical zone consists of thousands of minute, rounded bodies, the glomeruli,

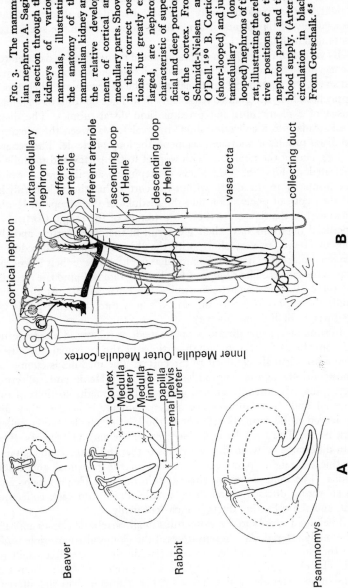

FIG. 3. The mammalian nephron. A. Sagittal section through the kidneys of various mammals, illustrating the anatomy of the mammalian kidney and the relative development of cortical and medullary parts. Shown in their correct positions, but greatly enlarged, are nephrons characteristic of superficial and deep portions of the cortex. From Schmidt-Nielsen and O'Dell.[190] B. Cortical (short-looped) and juxtamedullary (long-looped) nephrons of the rat, illustrating the relative positions of the nephron parts and the blood supply. (Arterial circulation in black.) From Gottschalk.[65]

B

juxtamedullary nephron

afferent arteriole

efferent arteriole

cortical nephron

ascending loop of Henle

descending loop of Henle

vasa recta

collecting duct

Inner Medulla | Outer Medulla | Cortex

A

Beaver

Cortex
Medulla (outer)
Medulla (inner)
renal pelvis
ureter
papilla

Rabbit

Psammomys

and greatly contorted tubules. The medullary zone consists of fine straight tubules packed tightly together. In order to discern further the anatomy of the kidney it is necessary to resort to more specialized anatomical techniques.

By various methods, such as teasing out of tissues fixed and macerated in concentrated acid, reconstruction of microscopic sections (montages) and so on, the anatomical relationships of the nephrons and their blood supply have been ascertained reasonably well. The nephrons of mammals consist of a glomerulus and proximal and distal tubules. The distal tubule leads into a collecting duct. Intercalated between the proximal and distal tubules is a straight segment, the loop of Henle. The general arrangement of the nephrons with respect to the cortex and medulla is illustrated in Fig. 3b. Two kinds of nephrons are illustrated which vary primarily in the depth within the cortex that their glomeruli lie and the depth of penetration into the medulla of their loops of Henle. Illustrated in the figure are the two extremes of the range. Cortical or superficial nephrons have their glomeruli in the outer cortex, and the loops of Henle are very short, with the thin segment much reduced. Juxtamedullary (i.e. next to the medulla) nephrons have their glomeruli deep in the cortex. Their loops of Henle penetrate well into the medulla and some of them reach to the tip of the renal papilla. At the renal papilla the nephrons (collecting ducts) empty into the renal pelvis via the ducts of Bellini (not shown).

In summary, generalizations can be made as follows. The glomeruli and convoluted (pars convoluta) portions of the proximal and distal tubules are virtually confined to the cortex. The medulla is composed almost entirely of the long and short loops of Henle and collecting ducts (plus, of course, the blood vessels). The straight portions of the proximal and distal tubules are also medullary. However, they are considered to be a functional part of the loop of Henle, the so-called thick limbs. The medulla is divided into inner and outer zones. The main difference between the two zones is that the outer zone contains the thick, straight (pars recta) portions of the proximal and distal tubules. The inner zone contains the thin limbs of Henle's loops and the collecting ducts. Several distal tubules drain into each collecting duct, and the collecting ducts branch repeatedly.

The blood supply to the glomerulus in all vertebrate classes appears to be solely arterial. An afferent (toward the glomerulus) arteriole leads into the Bowman's capsule, where it ramifies into a net-like capillary bed. The glomerular capillaries form into an efferent (away from the glomerulus) arteriole, which has a smaller diameter than the afferent arteriole. The efferent arteriole leads into a (peritubular) capillary network which surrounds the balance of the nephron. In general, the cortical efferent arterioles break up into the peritubular capillaries around the proximal and distal convoluted tubules. The juxtamedullary efferent arterioles supply the vasa recta of the medulla. The capillaries of the cortex and medulla drain into the renal vein.

As in other organs, there is a lymphatic system, i.e. a system of tortuous passages in the interstitium. There is some question as to whether or not the cortical regions of the kidney have a lymphatic system.[98] In animals which possess renal portal systems (birds, reptiles, amphibians and fishes), there is also an afferent venous supply to the tubules, or parts of the tubules. In birds there is some question as to whether the renal portal system does more than merely pass through the kidneys.

Chapter 2

Renal organs are part of the homeostatic system of animals, although their relative importance in homeostasis varies from group to group. All renal organs elaborate a fluid (primary urine) whose composition is varied by active and passive mechanisms. Whilst elaborating the urine renal organs carry on the following specific processes: fluid-volume regulation, adjustment of body fluid concentrations of inorganic ions and organic metabolites and elimination of actually or potentially toxic metabolites. Knowledge of the contribution of renal organs to the foregoing specific processes varies considerably between animal groups. It is known that in mammals the kidneys make an important contribution to all of the listed processes. Only fluid–volume regulation is yet known to be common to renal organs of non-mammals, probably reflecting the paucity of studies of such organs.

At all stages in the formation and elaboration of urine, fluid and solutes move across renal epithelia. In an attempt to avoid ambiguity in the use of terms which often plagues elementary accounts of solute and fluid movements, terms which will be used throughout the text will be defined here.

Terms of osmotic concentration

In many cases, fluid movement is due to differences in osmotic pressure on two sides of a membrane or epithelium. Since it is difficult to study pressure differences directly, those differences are inferred by the study of differences in the concentration of solutes which give rise to the pressure differences. Three terms are utilized to express concentration, namely, tonicity, molarity and molality. These terms often are used interchangeably; nevertheless, they have precise and different meanings.

The use of the term tonicity arises from studies of tissues isolated in artificial media. If tissues neither swelled nor shrank in an artificial medium, it was assumed that the tissue and medium had equal osmotic pressure or tension (tonus); that is, they were isotonic. In recent years, this somewhat pragmatic approach has given way to more precise methods of determining the osmotic pressure of tissues and biological fluids, methods deriving from an appreciation of the applicability of the 'laws' of ideal gases to solutes in solution.

One concept derived from the gas laws is that of molarity. One mole (i.e. 6.02×10^{23} molecules) of an 'ideal' (non-polar) gas, when confined to a litre volume at standard temperature and pressure, has sufficient kinetic energy to exert a pressure of 22.4 atmospheres. Certain modifications of the gas laws are necessary before they can be applied to solutes in solution. First, unlike gases, different solutes occupy different volumes. Therefore, it is necessary to standardize on weight rather than volume. One mole of solute dissolved in one kilogram of water became the standard and this is called a molal solution. All of the different manifestations of the effect on the energy of one kilogram of water caused by dissolution of one mole of solute in the water, osmotic pressure, elevation of the vapour pressure and boiling point, lowering of the freezing point, are the colligative properties of solutions. Any one can be calculated from measurement of any other.

Until recently, the term of choice for biologists has been molarity, since it is more convenient to measure the volumes of biological fluids. Concomitantly, concentrations have been expressed in terms of moles per litre ($M\ l^{-1}$). Where colligative properties such as freezing point have been measured, these usually have been expressed relative to a standard solution (e.g. freezing point $= X\ mM\ l^{-1}$ NaCl). However, it is becoming increasingly common to measure the colligative properties of biological solutions in terms of an absolute standard, such as the depression of the freezing (melting) point ($\Delta°C$). In such measurements it is necessary to express concentrations in terms of molality or moles per kilogram of water ($M\ kg^{-1}\ H_2O$).

A second modification of the gas laws necessary in order to apply them to solute solutions was to take into consideration the dissociation of solute molecules. Many solute molecules dissociate in water. One mole of solute in solution still contains 6.02×10^{23} molecules, but more than that number of particles may be present. Since the colligative properties of solute solutions depend upon the number of particles present, the energy of the solution will increase accordingly. A mole of solute which does not dissociate (e.g. glucose) has the same kinetic activity as about one-half mole of sodium chloride which dissociates almost completely into sodium and chloride ions. Therefore, a 0·5 molal solution of sodium chloride has the osmotic equivalence of a one molal solution of glucose. In order to express the osmotic equivalence of solute solutions, there is an increasing tendency to use the terms *osmo*larity and *osmo*lality. Two solutions which have the same number of osmotic equivalents are said to be isosmolar or isosmolal. Like the glucose and sodium chloride solutions mentioned above, such solutions may not be isomolar or isomolal. Measurement of the osmotic concentration of biological tissues and fluids usually involves the measurement of osmolar or osmolal concentrations. Rarely is the composition of the fluid sufficiently well known for an investigator to be able to compute molar or molal concentration from a measured colligative property.

The terms tonicity, molarity/molality and osmolarity/osmolality often are used with comparative prefixes: *iso* means 'equal to', *hypo* means 'less than', and *hyper* means 'greater than'.

Filtration, ultrafiltration and arterial filtration.

These three terms are used interchangeably, often giving rise to unnecessary confusion. In a strict sense, filtration is the process whereby fluid passes through a porous membrane (surface) driven by a differential in hydrostatic pressure across the membrane. Ultrafiltration results when the pores through which fluid moves restrict the passage of molecules too large to be in true solution (colloids). The word ultrafiltration was originally coined to describe filtration in the vertebrate glomerular kidney. It was thought that colloids do not pass through the glomerular filter so that ultrafiltration and glomerular filtration came to be synonymous. It is now known that colloids do pass through the glomerular filter; however, the term ultrafiltration has been retained and has come to be synonymous with arterial filtration (defined below).

The energy required to establish the hydrostatic pressure differential necessary for filtration may arise from at least two sources. First, the energy of the heart or contractile blood vessel may serve to 'press' fluid through the filtering surface from the blood space into the lumen of the renal organ. Secondly, the beat of cilia or flagella within the lumen of the renal organ may 'pull' fluid across the filtering surface. The first process, arterial filtration, is thought to exist in glomerular kidneys and in some invertebrate renal organs. The second process is thought to exist in invertebrates whose renal organs are protonephridia. Presumably the two processes differ only in the source of the energy which establishes the hydrostatic pressure difference.

Filtration may occur when the sum of the forces causing fluid to move out of the blood or body fluid space exceeds the sum of forces resisting such movement. Forces which resist filtration are the 'oncotic' pressure of the blood or body fluid and the general hydrostatic resistance of the tissues through which the filtered fluid must flow. Oncotic pressure is a term used to describe the sum of the osmotic pressure exerted by non-filtered solutes (colloids) and the general imbibatory (water-attracting) properties of colloids. Factors favouring filtration are, of course, blood or body fluid hydrostatic pressure and the oncotic pressure of the primary urine.

Filtration as a purely physical process is readily understood. However, the process which occurs in various renal organs is less readily understood, primarily because the nature of the filtering surfaces is, as yet, poorly defined.

Diffusion

Diffusion is the movement of substances from an area of high concentration to an area of low concentration. In biological systems diffusion often occurs through membranes or epithelia whose characteristics are incompletely known. Diffusive processes which occur in biological systems are only partially understood.

Active transport.

Filtration and diffusion may account for transmembrane or transepithelial solute and water movement. However, these passive processes cannot, by themselves, lead to the establishment of gradients of concentration. Concentration gradients may be attributed to passive membrane impermeability or the active metabolism of the cells. Wherever there is evidence that solutes or water move across membranes or epithelia against the concentration gradient, active transport may be suspected. However, before it can be confirmed that active transport is involved a number of criteria must be investigated.

Probably all cells have an **electrical gradient** across their membranes; the interior of the cells is negative relative to the exterior. The interior negativity is probably due to the presence within cells of large anions and negatively-charged proteins to which cell membranes are impermeable. Diffusible cations tend to move into cells to balance the negative charge; diffusible anions tend to move out of cells to balance the positive charge outside. The effect of large indiffusible anions and negatively-charged proteins on the diffusion of anions and cations is called the Donnan effect. Diffusible cations may become concentrated within cells or on the side of epithelia on which proteins are found. Diffusible anions may become concentrated on the side of membranes where proteins are absent, replacing, as it were, the indiffusible, negatively-charged solutes. The Donnan effect is a static effect and does not require cellular energy. In fact, it is demonstrated readily using artificial membranes (e.g. dialysis bags) which enclose protein solutions.

At equilibrium, the Donnan effect must exactly balance the diffusion force of the anions and cations. That is, cations which are being held on the negatively-charged side of the membrane will tend to diffuse down the concentration gradient and away from the negatively-charged side of the membrane. Similarly, anions wll tend to diffuse away, down the concentration gradient, from the positively-charged side of the membrane. The force required to exactly balance this diffusion force or pressure is described by the Nernst equation, which relates concentration (thermal activity) and electrical charge to the electromotive force (electrical potential) involved. A common working form of the Nernst equation for univalent ions is as follows:

$$E = -58 \log_{10} \frac{C_{in}}{C_{out}},$$

where E is the electromotive force in millivolts and C_{in} and C_{out} are the concentrations of the univalent ion on either side of the membrane.

The use of the Nernst equation can be illustrated as follows. The potassium concentration in the haemolymph and the lumen of the Malpighian tubules of an insect was found to be, respectively, $10\ mM l^{-1}$ and $100\ mM\ l^{-1}$. If this concentration difference represents an equilibrium condition, it should give rise to a potential difference across the Malpighian tubule epithelium of -58 millivolts [i.e. -58 ($\log_{10}$ of $100/10$), $= -58 \times 1$]. If the measured electrical potential difference is less than -58 millivolts, or if it is positive, then some process other than the Donnan equilibrium must be involved; that process may be active transport.

In order to overcome the electrical gradients across cellular and epithelial membranes, cellular energy must be expended. The energy expenditure required is minimal if the solute moving across the membrane is neutral. This is thought to be the reason why electrically-neutral solutes move more readily across membranes than do electrically-charged solutes of a similar size and shape.

Concentration gradients may arise by a number of mechanisms which are thought not to require cellular energy. The electrical gradient may give rise to concentration gradients. Additionally, because of their size, shape and chemical composition, some solutes penetrate biological membranes only with difficulty, resulting in a concentration gradient across the membrane. In general, lipid-soluble solutes penetrate membranes more readily than do water-soluble solutes of similar size and shape.

Concentration gradients for some readily diffusible solutes may arise through a process known as ionic or molecular 'trapping.' For example, dissolved ammonia gas is relatively non-polar and therefore very diffusible. Ammonia may diffuse into the lumena of renal organs where conditions may be more acidic than in the blood or cells. The acidic conditions cause hydration of the ammonia gas (NH_3) forming the less-diffusible ammonium ions (NH_4^+). A high concentration of ammonia may accumulate in ionic form on one side of a membrane or epithelium. A similar mechanism may account for the trapping of carbon dioxide as bicarbonate (HCO_3^-) in alkaline media. Steroids, being lipid-soluble, penetrate cell membranes readily. To counteract their tendency to diffuse across cell membranes, they may be conjugated to electrically-charged molecules. Steroids may therefore be 'trapped' in the kidney lumen by conjugation to proteins.

TABLE 1

Some commonly used inhibitor substances, their possible sites of action and effects.

Inhibitor	Probable action	Effect
COMPETITIVE INHIBITORS		
Arsenate	Competes with PO_4 for 'carrier'	Stops phosphate transport.
Benemid	Competes with organic acids for transport 'carrier' sites	Diminishes rate of organic acid (PAH, PSP) secretion
Phlorizin	Competes with glucose for transport 'carrier' sites	Stops glucose transport
OTHER INHIBITORS		
Copper ions	Block 'pores' in membranes	Stop movement of chloride
Cyanide (and Azide)	Inhibit cytochrome oxidase	Stop cell metabolism
Diamox	Inhibits carbonic anhydrase	Stops Na:H exchange; increases urinary HCO_3, K
2,4-Dinitrophenol	Stops oxidative phosphorylation	Slowly or rapidly stops cell metabolism (depending upon high-energy PO_4 reserves)
Iodoacetate	Inhibits conversion of glucose-6-PO_4 to pyruvate	Stops glycolysis
Ouabain	Inhibits Na, K activated adenosine triphosphatase	Stops sodium transport, fluid flow

Inhibition of active transport can be effected in a number of ways. Low temperature and anoxia both slow solute and fluid movements in many preparations. In addition, several chemical compounds exhibit inhibitory effects on active transport. Some of these and their possible mode of action are listed in Table 1.

Some chemical inhibitors directly inhibit enzyme reactions, others inhibit competitively. Competitive inhibition is thought to arise by a process where two or more solutes compete for the same transport mechanism (carrier site). Alternatively, the two compounds may compete for the same sources of energy within the cell. The effect is to diminish the transport rate of one or both solutes, depending upon the relative affinity of the transport mechanism for the solutes (see Fig. 15 p. 51) and the directness of access of the transport mechanism to the energy sources within the cell. Other chemical inhibitors as a group deprive the active transport mechanisms of their energy source. This may arise through a direct effect upon the carrier mechanism, as may occur in ouabain poisoning (Table 1). Alternatively, there may be an effect on the energy-supplying metabolic steps. The general inhibitor, 2,4-dinitrophenol, is thought to act by preventing phosphorylation in the oxidative phases of metabolism. Thus ouabain appears to deprive the carrier mechanism alone of its energy source, but the cells still function; dinitrophenol may deprive the cells of energy which poisons both cells and carrier mechanism.

Where such factors as electrical potential differences, differences in diffusibility or solubility and hydrostatic pressure can be ruled out, movement of solute and fluid across epithelia or cell membranes, almost by definition, is due to active transport. Where transepithelial fluid or solute movement can be inhibited by chemical inhibitors strong evidence for active transport exists, but lack of inhibition does not necessarily rule out active transport. The action of chemical inhibitors, with few exceptions, is not well understood.

Load-independent and load-dependent transport. Where it can be established that transport of a given solute is active, it can be shown that this transport is of two main kinds. The rate of transport of any solute, at least for a time, is dependent upon the amount (load) of solute available for transport. In many cases, the rate of active transport rises to a maximum as the load is increased (see curve C, Fig. 15, left). This maximum rate is termed the transport maximum or T_{max}. When the T_{max} is reached the concentrations of solute on either side of the transporting membrane become independent of each other. Thus the transport load is load independent. The simplest explanation of T_{max} is that a 'carrier' of some kind is involved in moving solute across membranes. It is envisaged that the carrier may become saturated; that is, that it may operate at a maximum rate, when the load of transportable solute exceeds a certain value.

In some systems, T_{max} is never reached within a non-deleterious or 'physiological' range of solute load. This is said to be load-dependent transport. If carriers are involved in load-dependent transport, presumably, they must be unsaturable.

Secretion and reabsorption

Secretion and reabsorption are general terms used to describe increases and decreases, respectively, in the concentrations or quantities of solutes and water. These terms imply that energy-requiring processes may cause changes in concentration or volume but the nature of the processes has not been established. Where an energy-requiring step is known to exist, the adjective 'active' often is used.

Clearance, clearance ratio, glomerular filtration rate and filtration fraction

By definition, clearance is the amount of plasma or body fluid cleared of a given substance in a known time, whether by filtration or secretion. The clearance is equal to the urine concentration (U) multiplied by the rate of blood flow (V) and divided by the plasma concentration (B) (i.e. clearance $= UV/B$). In the equation, the concentration terms cancel so that clearance is a rate (e.g. ml min^{-1}). If a substance is known not to be reabsorbed once it enters the urine, its clearance is equal to the rate of filtration or secretion.

Knowledge of function in many kidneys has been advanced by studies of inulin excretion by glomerular kidneys. Because inulin is filtered only, its clearance is equal to the rate of primary urine formation. Furthermore, since inulin is not reabsorbed after filtration, comparison of its concentration in the final urine with the concentrations of other compounds in the final urine may yield insight into events altering the concentrations of substances after they enter the urine. One way of making such comparisons is to calculate the clearance ratio. The urine: plasma ratio (U/P) for the substance under test (U_x/P_x) is divided by the U/P for inulin (U_i/P_i). If the compound is handled in the same way as inulin, the clearance ratio ($U_x/P_x \div U_i/P_i$) should be unity. If the clearance ratio is greater than one, secretion of the test substance is indicated. If the clearance ratio is less than one, reabsorption of the test substance may be indicated. This concept becomes inadequate when dealing with substances such as potassium, which may be filtered, secreted and reabsorbed. Furthermore, when a substance suffers restricted entry into the nephron lumen (say, because of its large size) the clearance ratio may be less than unity. In this case, however, it is not possible to tell precisely what events have occurred to alter its concentration by analysis of the final urine.

In the literature describing function of vertebrate kidneys, the terms 'glomerular filtration rate' and 'filtration fraction' are often encountered. Glomerular filtration rate (usually abbreviated to *GFR*) is a specialized usage of clearance. It is the clearance of compounds which are neither secreted nor reabsorbed; examples of such compounds are inulin, polyvinylpyrolidone (PVP), dextrans, polyfructosan (an inulin-like substance) and creatinine. Creatinine is secreted by some animals, but in others it is only filtered. The filtration fraction is that amount of a substance entering the glomerulus which is filtered. It can be estimated by measuring the concentration of the substance in the renal artery (pre-kidney plasma) and renal vein (post-kidney plasma). The amount of a substance, e.g. inulin, lost in passing through the kidney, is assumed to have been filtered; that is, it is the filtration fraction.

Techniques of study of renal organs

Concepts in any field are better understood even if only a rudimentary knowledge is possessed of the methods used to obtain the results upon which the concepts are based. Here attention will be focused upon a few techniques which have advanced understanding of renal function. These fall into two broad categories 'direct' and 'indirect'.

Direct methods are those in which all or a part of the renal organ is subjected to direct manipulation. Two such methods have had significant influence on our current interpretation of renal mechanisms. These are the micropuncture technique and various modifications of the perfusion technique.

The micropuncture technique. A micropipette is placed into the lumen of the kidney (Fig. 4A) and a small sample of fluid is withdrawn whilst flow in the lumen continues (free-flow), or is halted by blocking the lumen (stopped-flow). Usually the bore of the micropipettes is sufficiently small (2 to 50μ) to permit the lumenal fluid to rise into the pipette by capillarity. Placement of the micropipette requires the use of a micromanipulator, and the whole procedure is carried out during observation with the low to medium powers (10× to 100×) of a stereomicroscope.

Perfusion techniques. The kidney or parts of the kidney may be removed and bathed in an artificial medium, such as Ringer solution or serum (Fig. 24). Test substances are placed in the artificial medium and their rate of disappearance from the medium and/or the rate of their appearance in the fluid produced can be determined.

B

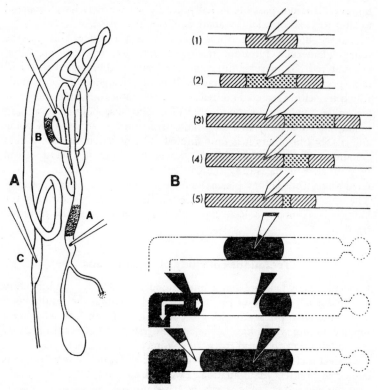

FIG. 4. **A.** Fluid collection by micropuncture from the early (A), middle (B) and late (C) proximal tubule of *Necturus*. The tubule is blocked (stippling) downstream from the puncture site. From Richards.[171] **B.** The split-droplet method of microperfusion. *Top:* Oil is injected into the lumen from a double-barrelled pipette (1). The droplet is split by injection of perfusion fluid (2), and more oil is injected to move the perfusion fluid from the puncture site (3). The rate of fluid reabsorption can be determined by photographic or visual measurements of the distance between the menisci taken at appropriate intervals (4, 5). *Bottom:* Where it is desired to recover the perfusion fluid, oil is injected into the lumen and split with perfusion fluid. At a site distal to the first pipette, a second pipette is inserted and oil injected to block the lumen. Fluid is recovered through the second pipette by injecting more oil from the first pipette. From Giebisch and Windhager.[60]

A specialization of the perfusion method is the stopped-flow microperfusion technique (Fig. 4B). An oil droplet is placed into the lumen of the renal organ, blocking it and halting lumenal fluid flow. Then perfusion fluid of known composition is introduced into the oil droplet, causing it to separate into two halves, which lie on either side of the perfusion fluid. After some time, the perfusion fluid may be recovered with another pipette and its contents analyzed for changes from the original composition. Alternatively, the rate of disappearance of the droplet can be determined by photographic or visual means.

Two indirect methods of study have significantly advanced knowledge of renal function. These are 'stop-flow' and 'renal-test-substance-injection' techniques.

The stop-flow technique. This technique has been used successfully only on a few animals. The animal is anaesthetized; the kidneys are exposed and one ureter or other distal part is catheterized. Flow of urine is stopped either by clamping the ureter or by applying a back pressure through the catheter. After a period of time, flow is resumed and the urine is collected in serial samples and analyzed.

The theory of the stop-flow technique is that changes in urine composition effected by various parts of the kidney will be intensified if the urine flow through them stops. The urine from the various parts of the nephrons can be identified in several ways. For example, after stopping flow, a substance which is known to be handled by one specific segment of the nephron may by infused into the renal artery: *Para*-amino hippurate is secreted solely by the proximal tubule of the mammalian nephron. Urine samples containing PAH therefore can be identified as coming from the proximal tubule; earlier samples come from regions more distal than the proximal tubule. To identify urine which has been formed after flow is restarted, inulin is infused into the renal artery during occlusion or just before flow is restarted.

The stop-flow technique is not without its problems. Since the nephrons of mammalian kidneys are of differing lengths (Fig. 3), there is often mixing of urine from different parts of the nephron. Also, it has been found recently that 'filtration' (inulin clearance) may continue for some minutes after the urine flow is stopped by ureteral clamping.

Injection of test substances. By far the commonest method of study of renal physiology is that of test-substance injection or perfusion. An enormous variety of compounds have been tested. Attention will be confined here to inulin and *para*-amino hippuric acid (PAH), both of which exhibit rather characteristic action on all animals thus far tested.

Inulin is a polysaccharide composed of an unknown number of fructose units. It has a molecular weight of about 5000. It is chemically stable in neutral or alkaline solutions, and it is not known to be metabolized by the cells or body fluid of any animal. Inulin is not normally taken up by the cells of the vertebrate kidney in appreciable amounts, yet it appears in the urine.[171,199] A reasonable conclusion from this evidence is that inulin is filtered, i.e. it enters the urine by a passive process not involving cellular uptake. The crucial proof of the filtration of inulin was provided by Richards,[171] who showed that the concentrations of inulin in the plasma and in the primary urine (glomerular fluid) were nearly identical. In recent years various investigators have published evidence of the entry of inulin into cells and its reabsorption from the urine. However, most of these discrepancies have been resolved satisfactorily by subsequent investigation.[209]

Para-amino hippuric acid is secreted by the vertebrate kidney. Secretion seems to be confined to the proximal tubule. The compound is composed of a benzene ring conjugated to an amino acid, glycine. In vertebrates, it is the end product of one of the main pathways by which amino acids are deaminated.

A very large number of molecules have renal clearance which are greater than simultaneously-determined inulin clearances. It is considered that these substances are secreted. In addition to PAH, the dye phenol red (phenolsulfonephthalein or PSP) is secreted by a wide variety of animals. *Para*-aminohippuric acid and PSP are acidic, and they appear to be secreted by a common pathway. Many organic bases are also secreted, and they appear to share a pathway different from that of the organic acids.

A further indirect method of study of renal function bears mentioning. Dyes are injected into various animals and analyses made of the organs that the dyes stain vitally. The results of these studies are difficult to interpret, since the physical properties of the dyes are as yet insufficiently known. However, the method has resulted in the identification of a large number or organs, tissues and cells which accumulate dyes. Possibly many of these accumulation sites are to be considered renal in function.

Of all the various methods of study of renal function, micropuncture and related techniques remain the most definitive. Richards' use of this method provided strong support for the filtration function of the glomerulus and quieted a controversy which had raged for nearly a century (see Chapter 3). Whereas the micropuncture technique has provided the least equivocal evidence for the function of several renal organs, it has drawbacks. First, it is tedious. In most cases a tiny pipette with a tip diameter of only a few microns must be placed accurately in the interior of the kidney. This requires a reasonably sophisticated (and expensive) micromanipulator. Secondly, because of their opacity or remoteness, not all renal organs or parts of renal organs are accessible for micropuncture. In most mammalian kidneys only a few surface nephrons are accessible. The remainder lie buried in the opaque interior of the kidney. The interior of the kidney may be exposed by removing portions, but this involves the risk that the tissue function thereby will be impaired.

Perhaps the greatest drawback to the micropuncture technique is the difficulty of analyzing the samples obtained. In most cases, the sample size can be measured in nannolitres (nl, 10^{-9} litres) or microlitres (μl or 10^{-6} litres). The small size of the samples requires fairly specialized analytical techniques which tend to be expensive, tedious or both. Nevertheless, methods have been devised for the satisfactory determination of many important parameters, osmotic pressure, inorganic ions and organic compounds (see reference 234).

Indirect methods are easier to apply than direct methods of renal study. Greater amounts of fluid can be collected during experimental periods which greatly facilitates analyses. Probably the greatest bulk of renal studies today are made in connexion with the clinical aspects of renal function or malfunction. Since these studies involve the least accessible mammal of them all, man, only indirect methods can be used.

Part 2: Function of Vertebrate Nephrons

Chapter 3

In 1842 Bowman demonstrated that the space which bears his name is contiguous with the nephron tubule. He injected coloured material into the renal corpuscle and noted that the colour spread into the tubule. Bowman speculated that the glomerulus is responsible for providing the water necessary to separate and dissolve materials eliminated by the tubule. In 1844, Ludwig published his now famous theory. He speculated that urine formation is brought about by a process of ultrafiltration in the glomerulus. That is, the arterial pressure 'presses' water and crystalloids from the blood plasma. The final urine results from the purely passive back diffusion of much of the water and some of the crystalloids into the blood spaces surrounding the tubule. The impetus for movement of fluid out of the tubule into the peritubular blood spaces is provided by plasma colloids which have been concentrated by the filtration process.

Ludwig's theory could not stand unaltered in the light of evidence acquired after its pronouncement. First, the histological appearance of parts of the tubule suggested abundant secretory activity by the cells. Secondly, passive back diffusion of water and crystalloids into the blood from the tubules could not result in a blood-hypertonic urine, yet such a urine was produced by mammals.

In the latter part of the 19th century, the experiments and arguments of Heidenhain helped to re-establish the dominance of the secretion theory of Bowman. He showed that the dye indigo carmine became concentrated in the tubule; apparently the dye does not appear in the renal corpuscle. Further, he estimated that the amount of blood which must be filtered to account for all of the urea excreted by a man in a day was in excess of the amount of blood that flows through the kidney in a day. Finally, he reasoned that urine flow was most affected by the velocity of blood flow through the kidney, rather than the pressure of the blood. It would be expected that the rate of blood flow would influence the opportunity of the cells to remove materials from the blood, whereas the pressure of the blood would not necessarily influence removal.

Early in the 20th century the Ludwig theory was again resurrected, largely because of experiments on the effects of altering glomerular and ureteral pressures on urine flow. In 1917, Cushny published a theory in which urine formation was seen as a process of filtration in the glomerulus followed by reabsorption by the tubules. This logical conclusion of several decades of argument stands as the basis of the modern theory of urine formation.

For some eighty years after Bowman's original speculations, the pendulum swung between the secretion theory of Bowman and Heidenhain and the filtration-reabsorption theory of Ludwig and Cushny. Both of these theories agreed that the glomerulus is important to urine formation, but they presented different views of the importance of its function.

In the first half of the 20th century experimental evidence began to accumulate which favoured a filtration role for the glomerulus. Investigations of intraglomerular arterial pressures and renal venous pressures indicated that filtration is possible. Nevertheless, the absence of direct evidence for filtration left considerable room for doubt. However, in 1924, Wearn and Richards[227] published analyses of fluid taken directly from the glomerulus. The analyses showed clearly that glomerular fluid conforms closely in composition to a plasma filtrate. This study established the filtration hypothesis in a strong position.

The overall function of glomerular nephrons

The generalized pattern of urine formation and elaboration derived from micropuncture studies of amphibians and mammals is shown in Fig. 5. Not shown is the contribution of medullary components of mammalian nephrons which will be discussed separately (Chapter 6). Briefly, the amphibian and mammalian nephrons adhere to the same basic plan. In both, a protein-free fluid, derived from the plasma, enters the uriniferous (Bowman's) space of the glomerulus. In the proximal tubule this fluid is modified by the reabsorption of sodium, potassium, chloride, water, glucose and a host of other solutes not shown. In some animals (e.g. *Necturus*, mammals) urea is also reabsorbed, but in frogs[171] urea appears to be secreted. In all vertebrates studied thus far, except hagfish,[158] phenol red is secreted in the proximal tubule, indicating the ubiquity of the organic-acid secreting mechanism in that segment. In mammals and probably in amphibians, hydrogen ion is secreted into the proximal tubule. The lumenal contents become very slightly acid (pH = 6·88) in mammals, but not in amphibians. In both mammals and amphibians the tubule fluid in the distal tubule is normally slightly acid.

In mammals, the tubule fluid: plasma ratio (TF/P) for inulin in the late proximal tubule is about three, indicating that about two-thirds of the water in the original filtrate has been reabsorbed. In the amphibian the end proximal TF/P for inulin is about 1·5, indicating that only about one-third of the filtered water is reabsorbed in the proximal tubule. The fluid (i.e. water plus solutes) which is reabsorbed in the proximal tubule is isosmotic or nearly isosmotic with the plasma. This is indicated by the fact that the TF/P for osmotic pressure in the late proximal tubule is still nearly one.

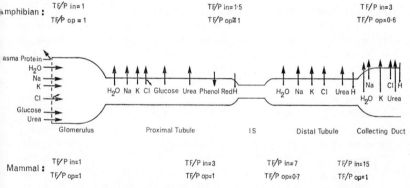

FIG. 5.   Net movements of water and various solutes in the nephrons of an amphibian (*Necturus*) and a mammal (rat). Not shown are the Henle's loops of mammals (see Fig. 20).

The distal tubule is the site of dilution of the urine, even in mammals where the final urine is usually much more concentrated than the plasma. Sodium, potassium, chloride and urea are all reabsorbed in the distal tubule, except that in frogs urea appears not to be reabsorbed distally. There appears to be secretion of potassium and hydrogen ion in the distal tubule of both amphibians and mammals. The fluid which is reabsorbed in the early distal tubule is hyperosmotic to the plasma, as indicated by the fact that the TF/P for osmotic pressure falls below unity. In amphibians, hyperosmotic reabsorption continues in the collecting duct (and probably the bladder) because the final urine may be quite dilute. In mammals, the fluid in the late distal tubule becomes isosmotic to the plasma. Of course, in the medullary portions of the collecting duct the tubule fluid may become much more concentrated than the general blood plasma.

The foregoing description is very generalized and describes conditions in the 'normal' animal. Both mammals and amphibians (apparently all animals) exhibit states of diuresis or anti-diuresis. Diuresis is a state of rapid urine flow. Two general kinds of diuresis are recognized. Osmotic diuresis results when the plasma levels of osmotically-active substances are elevated by injection or infusion. It is thought to be due to the retention of fluid in the lumen of the nephron due to an increase in amounts of osmotically active substances in the plasma filtrate. Water diuresis results from the lowering of the osmotic pressure of the plasma due to excessive intake of water. It is thought to be due to a phenomenon similar to osmotic diuresis except that there is an increase in the rate of filtration (GFR). The increased GFR speeds the rate of flow through the nephrons and thereby diminishes the time in which reabsorption of solutes can take place.

The degree of osmotic diuresis induced by increased levels of plasma solutes depends upon the nature of the solute. For example, if a solute such as mannitol, which is not reabsorbed from the tubule after filtration, is present, the diuresis is more severe than if the substance (e.g. sodium chloride) is reabsorbable.

Anti-diuresis is a state where meagre urine flow occurs. Mammals are normally anti-diuretic in that their urine is usually at least as concentrated as the plasma. As indicated by urine: plasma ratios for inulin as high as 700, anti-diuresis in mammals is accomplished by the reabsorption of water (as well as most of the solutes) from the urine. The ability to withdraw water from the urine is by no means unique to mammals or even to terrestrial vertebrates. Amphibians are known to be able to withdraw over 90% of the filtered water from the urine (i.e. the inulin $U/P \simeq 30$).

With this brief and very generalized introduction to the functions of the glomerular nephron, let us now examine in some detail the mechanisms involved in the formation and elaboration of the urine. These are, filtration, reabsorption, secretion and urine concentration.

Chapter 4

In Ludwig's view, the glomerulus acts as a mechanical barrier to the passage of large molecules. In recent years other views have been advanced which see the 'filter' as a selective membrane; selection is based on the chemical nature of plasma solutes as well as their size. One concept that has not altered appreciably since Ludwig's original hypothesis is the view that arterial pressure (i.e. the heart) is the energy source for filtration.

Ultrastructure of the glomerulus

The vertebrate glomerulus was one of the first structures to be investigated when the electron microscope came into wide-spread use after World War II. It was hoped that the accumulated physiological evidence for pores would be verified once and for all by morphological evidence. Unfortunately, this hope has yet to be realized.

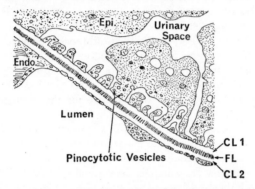

FIG. 6.   Ultrastructure of the glomerulus of a mammal. The bases of the capillary endothelial cells (Endo.) and visceral epithelial cells of the Bowman's capsule (Epi.) are embedded in cement layers (CL 1 and CL 2). Between the cement layers is a fibrous layer (FL). The capillary lumen (lumen) is in close approximation to the urinary space of the Bowman's capsule. Between the digitations of the bases of the epithelial cells are fine membranes. Pinocytotic vesicles are seen in both the capillary endothelial and visceral epithelial cells.

The relationship of the glomerular capillaries and the visceral (internal) layer of Bowman's capsule is shown in Fig. 6. The endothelium of the glomerular capillaries is closely applied to the epithelium of the visceral layer of the Bowman's capsule. The thin portion of the endothelial cells appears to have a porous or fenestrated structure. The diameters of the fenestrae range from 500 to 1000Å; they appear to be covered over with an exceedingly thin membrane, although the existence of this membrane is disputed. The visceral layer of Bowman's capsule consists of epithelial cells which have foot processes (hence they are called 'podocytes'). The foot processes or pedicels are partially embedded in the basement membrane at the bases of the cells. The podocytes have relatively large channels at their bases which are part of the uriniferous space. Where they meet the basement membrane the foot processes interdigitate; in close proximity to the basement membrane adjacent foot processes may be only 200 to 300Å apart. Here again, there appears to be a thin membrane covering the spaces between the foot processes.

Podocytes exhibit pinocytotic activity at their bases, and commonly their apical regions are filled with large vacuoles. In well-fixed material, these vacuoles can be seen as membrane-bound bodies (see frontispiece).

The space between the capillary endothelial cells and the podocytes is occupied by a basement membrane which resolves into three layers under the high magnification of the electron microscope. There are two cement layers, and an intermediate fibrous layer which gives the appearance of a felt mat. Some investigators claim that the fibres of this layer are the true filters; that there are spaces between the fibres whose diameters can be altered. However, this claim is refuted by other investigators who have found no evidence for the existence of such spaces.

The ultrastructure of the glomerulus appears to be fairly uniform throughout the vertebrates. The major differences between the various classes are seen in the height of the cells and the extent of the capillary and visceral epithelia. In mammals the visceral epithelial cells are rather squat and both the capillary and visceral epithelial layers are extensive. In lower vertebrates the visceral epithelial layers are less extensive. In birds many of the glomeruli become invaded with connective tissue, suggesting that bird nephrons are approaching the aglomerular condition.[95]

The pressures available for filtration

Measurement of pressure within the glomerular capillaries has proved to be technically very difficult. However, most indirect studies (see references 41, 234) bear out the following proposition: forces tending to facilitate fluid movement out of the glomerular capillaries (arterial pressure, oncotic pressure of the filtrate) are in excess of forces tending to keep fluid in the glomerular capillaries (oncotic pressure of the blood plasma, tissue resistance).

Richards and Plant[171] found that under conditions of constant blood flow, urine flow from the kidney of the rabbit increased whenever renal blood pressure was increased. This kind of experiment contradicted Heidenhain's contention that urine flow is related to blood flow and not blood pressure. Increase of blood pressure was effected by methods known to cause contraction of the renal arterial musculature (vasoconstriction): stimulation of vasoconstrictor nerves, addition of adrenalin to the perfusing blood, gentle constriction of the renal vein. The results of these experiments suggested that the vasoconstrictor effects occurred within the glomerular blood supply.[171] The most definitive proof of this suggestion came from studies in which glomeruli of frogs were visualized directly. Addition of adrenalin to blood perfusing frogs' kidneys caused enlargement of the glomerular capillary tuft within the renal capsule. This could be due only to the constriction of the efferent vessel of the glomerular capillary tuft. Subsequent to these experiments it was learned that the efferent vessel of the glomerular capillaries is an arteriole; thus its walls possess a musculature and are capable of contraction. These experiments provided indirect evidence that urine flow and intra-glomerular pressures are related.[171]

In other investigations attempts were made to quantify the pressures found within the various parts of the kidney. Studies have been made on the effect on urine flow of lowering the pressure in the glomerular capillaries or increasing the pressure of the interstitium. In mammals, urine flow ceases at a glomerular capillary pressure of about 36 mm Hg. This pressure still exceeds the colloid osmotic pressure of the plasma (25 mm Hg). Therefore, the resistance of the interstitial fluid may be as high as 11 mm Hg. The pressure normally available for filtration is probably considerably higher than 36 mm Hg, since filtration presumably stops at that pressure. The pressure drop between the glomerular capillaries and the renal artery is such that the pressure in the capillaries is about 60% of that in the artery. Therefore, at normal blood pressures of 90 to 100 mm Hg (systolic) the capillary hydrostatic pressure should be in the order of 60 mm Hg.[199]

Because of their more accessible glomeruli, it has heen possible to measure directly the pressure within the glomerular capillaries of the frog. Hayman[76] found that the glomerular capillary pressure in frogs averages $20 \cdot 2 \pm 6 \cdot 8$ cm H_2O. The colloid osmotic pressure of the blood plasma in frogs averages about 10 cm H_2O. Therefore, depending upon the interstitial resistance, there may be a net pressure of up to 10 cm H_2O to effect filtration.

If the filtration hypothesis is correct, the fluid which is expressed into the uriniferous space in the glomerulus should resemble a plasma ultrafiltrate: that is, blood plasma less plasma colloids. To test this hypothesis, Richards and his coworkers[171] began studies which have become classic. They removed samples of fluid from the glomerulus by micropuncture and analyzed them by colourimetric and other means. The results of these analyses are shown in Fig. 7. The composition of the glomerular fluid is very similar to that of the plasma, except that glomerular fluid has a higher concentration of chloride than plasma and contains only slight traces of protein. The results of glomerular fluid analyses were consistent with the filtration hypothesis, the elevated chloride concentrations possibly being due to the Donnan effect. That is, chloride ions would tend to diffuse into the glomerular fluid to balance an anion deficit caused by diminished protein concentration.

The inulin concentrations in glomerular fluid and plasma were approximately equal. This observation took on special significance for the proof of the filtration hypothesis. It indicated that a molecule of some size could move freely from the plasma to the glomerular fluid, which could only mean that smaller molecules move by an identical process: filtration.

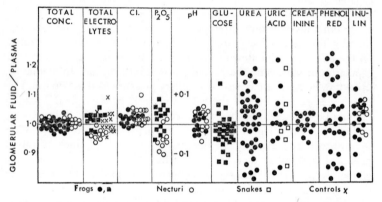

FIG. 7.   Concentration ranges of a variety of metabolites in glomerular fluid relative to the concentrations in the plasma. From Richards.[171]

Further experiments were performed in which oxygenated frog Ringer solution containing proteins was perfused through the renal artery. The smaller of the proteins, egg albumen (molecular weight $\simeq$ 45 000) was found in the glomerular fluid in amounts just a little less than in the perfusion fluid. No trace of the larger protein, horse serum albumen (molecular weight $\simeq$ 70 000), was found in the glomerular fluid. These results seemed to indicate that the glomerular filter is permeable to a molecule of 20Å radius (egg albumen), but it is impermeable to a molecule of 30 to 35Å radius (horse serum albumen). With these elegant and definitive experiments Richards and his colleagues established the filtration hypothesis in a virtually unassailable position. In fact, the filtration hypothesis is so firmly entrenched that students can be forgiven for being ignorant of the existence of an alternative hypothesis.

The results of mammalian micropuncture studies have confirmed and elaborated those obtained in studies of amphibians. Significantly, it has been shown that fairly large amounts of protein are present in the glomerular fluid of some mammals, notably the rat. However, in other mammals, such as dogs[5] very little protein is found in the glomerular fluid.

Permeability of the glomerular 'filter'

It is likely that pressure sufficient to effect filtration exists in the glomerular capillaries. However, until the characteristics of the filtering surface are known, it is not possible to define the characteristics of the filtration process in precise terms. Several studies have been made of the permeability of capillaries to molecules of various sizes. Permeability has been studied also in relation to the chemical composition of the permeant molecules. Most of these studies have been made on capillaries of tissues such as muscle, which are more accessible than are glomerular capillaries.

Studies of membrane permeability

It is known that natural membranes are composed of lipid and protein components. As particles penetrate natural membranes they must pass through areas whose chemical composition varies from their own. There may be at least two pathways through which particles may move passively across natural membranes. First, they may diffuse through the substance of the membrane. Second, they may pass through fluid-filled holes or pores in the membrane.

Pathway one: the ability of particles to pass through the substance of natural membranes depends upon their solubility (diffusibility) in lipids. Lipid-solubility, in turn, depends upon the number and disposition of electrical charges (polarity) of the particles. The less polar the particle, the more lipid soluble it is (see reference 41).

Pathway two: many biologically-important substances are highly polar and therefore have a very poor lipid solubility. However, they have a correspondingly high water solubility. Many polar substances (e.g. ions, water, amino acids) are able to penetrate natural membranes more rapidly, in fact, than their solubility in lipids would suggest is possible. This has led to the proposal that natural membranes contain water-filled pores through which water and water-soluble substances may move.

Numerous studies have been made of the theoretical and experimental aspects of the movement of dissolved particles through membranes (see references 40, 41, 46 and Chapter 12). However, applicability of various studies to the permeability of the glomerular filter will be the major concern here. Pappenheimer, Renkin and Borrerro[143] studied the permeability of capillaries in the isolated hind limb of the cat. Substances ranging in size from sodium chloride to haemoglobin were perfused into the blood supply to the hind limb. The rate of loss of the substances from the plasma permitted calculations of the permeability of the capillaries for each of the substances under test. The capillaries were most permeable to sodium chloride and impermeable to haemoglobin. From the calculated permeability and knowledge of the diffusibility of the test substances in water, it was possible to compute the area of pores necessary to account for the permeability of the capillaries to each substance. This theoretical pore area was called the 'restricted pore area' and was defined as the pore area necessary to permit free passage of each substance across the capillary wall. The restricted pore area ranged from zero for haemoglobin to 0·10 cm^2 per gram of muscle for sodium chloride. The restricted pore area describes the actual pore area only for small molecules, such as sodium chloride and water. Thus the actual pore area of the capillaries was 0·10 cm^2 per gram of muscle. Assuming that all of the sodium chloride (or water) passing through the capillaries diffused unrestricted through pores, the area required would amount to only about 0·15 % of the total capillary area.

The size of the pores which would be consistent with the observed permeability to water and the calculated restricted pore area of water was estimated. The 'effective pore radius' thus estimated was 30·5Å, assuming uniform, cylindrical pores. From these studies, it was concluded that the pores in the capillaries are sufficiently large to permit most plasma molecules smaller than proteins to pass.

Wallenius[225] studied the excretion of dextrans of varying molecular weights in an effort to characterize the permeability of the glomerular surface. Dextrans are polyglucosides which are synthesized in molecular sizes ranging from a few thousand to several million by certain bacteria when cultured in sucrose solutions. They can be separated or hydrolyzed into fractions containing different molecular weight ranges. In dogs, increasing molecular size brings about diminished clearance of dextrans (Fig. 8a). There was no sharp cut-off point above which clearance was halted and below which clearance was 100 %. On the contrary, clearance was diminished gradually the higher the molecular weight of the dextran, resulting in a sigmoid curve. In normal mammals the highest molecular weight dextran which could be detected in the urine varied from about 38 000 to 46 000, depending upon the species. Animals which were excreting protein in the urine (proteinuric) were able to clear much larger dextran molecules. In some strains of laboratory rats, proteinuria is a 'normal' condition. The largest molecular weight dextran which could be detected in the urine of these rats was about 63 000.

Dextrans are filtered much more readily than are proteins of similar (Einstein-Stokes) diffusion radii (Fig. 8b). Haemoglobin and serum albumen have diffusion radii of 30·5Å and 32·5Å, respectively. Clearance of similar-sized molecules of dextran is 60 to 70% of the glomerular filtration rate. Haemoglobin does not appear in the urine unless the blood concentration is elevated above about 100 mg per 100 ml. When haemoglobinuria occurs, the clearance does not exceed 13% of the

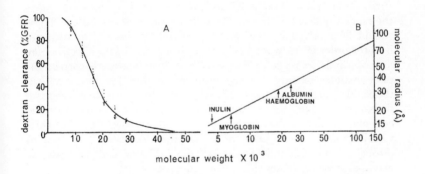

FIG. 8.   A. Renal clearance of dextrans relative to their molecular weights. B. Relationship between molecular weight and size (diffusion radii in Å) of dextrans. Arrows indicate the molecular weight : molecular size relationships of inulin and various proteins. Redrawn from Wallenius.[225]

glomerular filtration rate (references in 225). It is clear from this and other studies that charged particles (e.g. proteins) less readily enter the urine than do relatively uncharged molecules such as dextrans.

Wallenius' detection methods for dextrans were insensitive relative to methods used recently.[73] Radioactive dextran and polyvinylpyrolidone (PVP) molecules as large as c. 60Å molecular radius could be detected in the urine of rabbits. Molecules larger than about 24Å radius were subjected to a rapidly diminished clearance, however. Molecules no larger than 24Å radius were cleared freely. Thus the curve relating molecular size to glomerular permeability took on the sigmoid shape seen in Fig. 8a.

Capillaries, particularly glomerular capillaries, exhibit a phenomenon known as 'molecular sieving*. The permeability of the capillaries for particles of a given size diminishes the more rapid is the rate of fluid movement across the capillary. In terms of the pore hypothesis, this may be due to the following: in order that a particle may pass through a pore, it must not strike the edge; therefore, the faster the rate of movement through the pore, the greater will be the likelihood that even very small particles passing through large pores will strike the pore edge and be retarded.[142]

Non-kinetic studies of membrane permeability

The pore hypothesis of the permeation of membranes (particularly capillary membranes) by molecules is subject to several criticisms. First, electron micrographs fail to reveal pores whose sizes are within the range predicted by the studies of Pappenheimer and others. These should be resolved by the electron microscope since their diameter is in the order of 60 to 100Å. However, if analyses of the effective pore area of capillaries made by Pappenheimer[143] and others is correct, the pore area may be only an insignificant proportion (less than 0·2 %) of the capillary area. The chances of seeing a pore in an electron micrograph therefore would be remote. Nevertheless, large objects such as bacterial cells and colloidal carbon can penetrate capillary walls.[41] Furthermore, visualization of the passage of some large molecules (e.g. globin) through glomerular and other capillaries indicates that they pass as macro-aggregates, rather than dispersed molecules.[130]

It has been suggested that the passage of molecules across capillary membranes is a diffusion process. The entire capillary membrane may be permeable to water. Penetration of the membrane by other molecules would be dependent upon their diffusibility in the material of which the membrane is composed. The diffusion pathway may have a gel-like structure.[36] If formation of glomerular or capillary filtrate is a diffusion process, then the hydrostatic pressure in the capillaries would exert only a concentrating effect, increasing the rate of diffusion. However, it would be necessary for capillaries to have only a few pores in order that fluid movement across them be more rapid than by diffusion[142] (see chapter 12).

The fibrous structure of the middle layer of the glomerular basement membrane (Fig. 6) suggests that it may be composed of gelated material

---

* Molecular sieving is a dynamic, rather than a static effect. It is a term commonly and incorrectly applied when the more appropriate term, 'molecular filter' should be used. It is not correct to call a structure a molecular sieve unless the passive permeability of that structure for a given molecular species varies inversely with the rate of fluid flow through the structure.

(mucopolysaccharide). The porosity of the glomerulus might then depend upon the degree of cross-linkage of the gel. Thus the basement membrane may function as a molecular filter in a manner analogous to commercially-prepared gels, such as 'Sephadex'. The extent of cross-linkage between gel molecules determines the size of the spaces within gels. The size of the spaces determines the distance into the matrix of the gel that different-sized molecules can penetrate. Thus water and inorganic ions can occupy the smallest of the spaces in any particular gel; large molecules are excluded to a greater extent depending upon their size.

If the basement membrane of the glomerulus is a gelated molecular filter, the extent of cross-linking may vary with the physiological state of the animal. For example, in a disease state known as the 'nephrotic syndrome,' the glomerular basement membrane thickens. At the same time plasma proteinuria occurs. The proteinuria (and basement-membrane thickening) may result from a lessened extent of cross-linking in the basement-membrane.[82]

Movement of high-molecular-weight compounds across glomerular membranes has been followed by electron microscopy. Menefee and Mueller,[130] for example, have demonstrated that the protein, globin, passes as macroaggregates. The aggregates appear to enter the capillary endothelial cells by phagocytosis; they then cross the basement membrane and become 'lodged' against the membranes closing the fenestrae between adjacent foot processes of the podocytes. The podocytic membranes may be displaced by the globin aggregates, but there is no evidence that the basement membrane proper is displaced.

Menefee and Mueller[130] suggest that the basement membrane is the site of selection of molecules which pass the glomerular barrier. They argue that if the basement membrane were a rigid structure with fixed pores, aggregates as large as globin would either pile up on the endothelial side of the membrane or they would not pass at all. The basement membrane may act as a diffusion barrier to molecules which are soluble within the matrix of the membrane. In other instances (e.g. globin aggregates), the membrane may act as a 'thixotropic' gel (i.e. a gel which solates when pressure is applied to it.) The stability of gels depends upon the relative abundance of strong (covalent) and weak (electrostatic) bonds within the gel structure. Menefee and Mueller suggest that the gel structure of the glomerular basement membrane is relatively unstable. It may allow diffusion of particles without alteration of its structure. However, when an indiffusible aggregate apposes the gel, the gel liquifies locally, permitting the aggregate to pass.[130]

Palade[138] considers that fluid and dissolved solutes may cross capillary endothelial cells by a modified form of pinocytosis. The selection of the kinds of molecules and particles which will pass through the basement membrane is exercised by the capillaries.

In the foregoing we have attempted to outline what we consider to be some of the more interesting aspects of the modern interpretation of glomerular function. It is clear that we have still a long way to go before a complete understanding of the process we now call filtration is reached.

Variation in glomerular function

Glomeruli vary considerably in their rate of function. For example, in frogs, variations in the GFR of the kidneys are due to variations in the numbers of functioning glomeruli.[171] Horster and Thurau[79] studied the GFR of superficial (cortical) and juxtamedullary nephrons in the kidneys of rats. The rats were fed on diets low or high in sodium content. A high-sodium diet increases the rate of sodium excretion in the urine. A low sodium diet has the opposite effect. Timed collections of measured volumes of tubule fluid were made by micropuncturing the proximal and distal segments of cortical nephrons or the ascending and descending thin limbs of Henle's loops of juxtamedullary nephrons. The tubule fluid : plasma ratios for polyfructosan were also determined. From the rate of tubule fluid flow and the TF/P ratios for polyfructosan, it was possible to calculate the GFR of individual nephrons. The results are summarized in the upper part of Table 2. When the sodium load on the kidney is low (and sodium reabsorption from the urine is intensified), the GFR of individual juxtamedullary nephrons is higher than the GFR of individual superficial nephrons. When the sodium load on the kidneys is high (and sodium reabsorption from the urine is diminished) the GFR of the superficial nephrons exceed that of the juxtamedullary nephrons.

The rat kidney contains about 30 000 fairly uniform glomeruli.[79] Using the data summarized in Table 2 it was possible to calculate the total numbers of superficial and juxtamedullary nephrons in the rat kidney as follows:

$$GFR_{\text{Juxta.}} \times X + GFR_{\text{cort.}} \times 30\ 000 - X = GFR_{\text{total}}.$$

By calculation there appears to be about 6700 nephrons of the juxtamedullary type and 23 300 nephrons of the cortical type in the rat kidney. The proportion of juxtamedullary nephrons (i.e. about 22% of the total) agrees reasonably well with independently made morphological studies (Table 5). The data in Table 2 and the knowledge of the numbers of nephrons of each type permitted an estimate to be made of

TABLE 2

Glomerular filtration rates (GFR) of whole kidney and individual superficial and juxtamedullary nephrons in the laboratory rat and the sand rat (Psammomys). The GFR of laboratory rats was determined whilst the animals were fed on a diet high or low in sodium. The GFR of Psammomys was determined during saline infusion. Data on the laboratory rat from Horster and Thurau[79]. Data on Psammomys from de Rouffignac and Morel.[185]

	LABORATORY RAT	
	Low sodium diet	High sodium diet
Superficial nephron GFR (nl min^{-1} gm kidney weight)	23·5 ± 6·4	38·1 ± 11·3
Juxtamedullary nephron GFR (nl min^{-1} gm kidney weight)	58·2 ± 13·6	16·5 ± 6·6
Whole kidney GFR (ml min^{-1} gm kidney weight)	0·94 ± 0·16	1·01 ± 0·24
	PSAMMOMYS	
		Saline infusion
Superficial nephron GFR (nl min^{-1} per kidney)		9
Juxtamedullary nephron GFR (nl min^{-1} per kidney)		21·4

the contribution of nephrons of each type to the total *GFR* under high and low sodium loads.

When rats were maintained on a low sodium diet, the total *GFR* of the superficial glomeruli was $23\,300 \times 23\cdot5 \times 10^{-6}$ or 0·55 ml min^{-1} gm kidney weight. Since the total kidney *GFR* was 0·94 ml min^{-1} gm kidney weight, the superficial glomeruli filtered about 58% of the total filtrate. When rats were maintained on a high sodium diet the total *GFR* of the superficial glomeruli was $23\,300 \times 38\cdot1 \times 10^{-6}$ or 0·89 ml min^{-1} gm kidney weight. The total kidney *GFR* was 1·0 ml min^{-1} gm kidney weight, so that the superficial glomeruli filtered about 88% of the total filtrate.

In the laboratory rat at least, a high sodium load with its intensified sodium excretion is mediated by superficial nephrons. Low sodium loads with their concomitant low sodium loss in the urine are mediated by the juxtamedullary nephrons. The factors which control changes in the *GFR* observed in laboratory rats are unknown.

In the sand rat (*Psammomys*) the *GFR* of deep (juxtamedullary) nephrons exceeded that of superficial nephrons during sodium diuresis (Table 2). However, the glomeruli of nephrons which lie deep in the cortex are considerably larger than the glomeruli of superficial nephrons. Therefore, the results shown in Table 2 may only reflect a large difference in the filtering surfaces of superficial and deep glomeruli.[185]

Chapter 5

Reabsorption by the nephron tubule

Subsequent to filtration, fluid flows out of the proximal tubule lumen into the surrounding (peritubular) capillaries. Simultaneously, glucose and most of the sodium, potassium and chloride disappear from the tubule fluid. The final urine of most vertebrates is remarkably low in sodium and chloride. Figure 9 illustrates changes which occur in the concentrations of major constituents of the tubule fluid in the nephron of *Necturus*. With exceptions which will be discussed below, these changes are comparable both quantitatively and qualitatively to those seen in mammals.

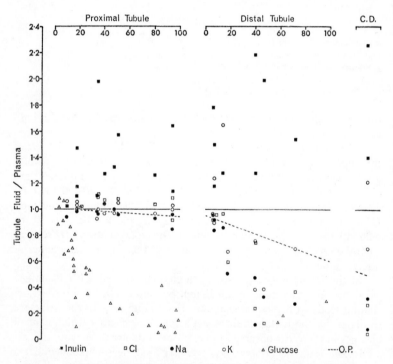

FIG. 9.   Tubule fluid : plasma ratios for inulin, osmotic pressure, glucose, sodium, potassium and chloride in various parts of the nephron of *Necturus*. The numbers beneath the designations 'proximal tubule' and 'distal tubule' refer to the parts of the nephrons (as a percentage of the total length of the segment) from which the samples were taken. Glucoes data from Richards.[171] The other data from Bott.[26]

Present evidence suggests that two mechanisms act to bring about the changes illustrated in Fig. 9. The first is that originally proposed by Ludwig: fluid reabsorption is a passive process. The colloid concentration of plasma passing into the peritubular capillaries rises due to filtration of water and non-colloids in the glomerulus. The oncotic pressure of the colloids attracts water across the tubule epithelium and small dissolved solutes accompany the water. The second mechanism bringing about the changes in concentration of water and solutes in the tubules is an active process. One solute, sodium, is actively transported across the tubule epithelium and water and small dissolved solutes follow passively.

Fluid reabsorption

The inulin TF/P values in Fig. 5 indicate that from one-third to two-thirds of the glomerular filtrate is reabsorbed in parts of the proximal tubule which are accessible to micropuncture. In mammals, there is evidence that in the inaccessible part of the proximal tubule, the inulin TF/P may rise to about four. The preponderance of fluid appears to be reabsorbed in the proximal tubules. Therefore, studies of fluid reabsorption have concentrated on that part of the nephron.

Proximal tubules of *Necturus* have been perfused with isosmotic sodium chloride solutions containing albumen.[229] The colloid osmotic pressure (COP) of the perfusion fluid was 15 cm H_2O, which is about one and one-half times the COP of the general plasma ($\simeq$ 10 cm H_2O). Under these experimental conditions, 15% of the perfusion fluid was reabsorbed by the tubules. When the tubule lumen was perfused with isosmotic sodium chloride solutions lacking colloid, 27% of the microperfusate was reabsorbed.[186] This amount of reabsorption was roughly comparable to that which occurs in unperfused tubules. The fluid which was reabsorbed from the lumen of the proximal tubule during microperfusion experiments was isosmotic to the plasma since the concentration of fluid remaining in the tubule was not changed. When the inhibitors, ouabain and 2,4-dinitrophenol (Table 1) were added to the perfusion fluid, fluid reabsorption was reduced to about one-third normal. Since fluid reabsorption occurred despite a presumably unfavourable colloid (albumen) concentration gradient and it was depressed by inhibitors of sodium transport and cellular metabolism, it was suggested that an active process must be involved.

In further experiments the sodium chloride concentration of the microperfusate was varied whilst the osmotic concentration was kept equal to that of the general plasma (about 100 mEq l^{-1}) with mannitol. Mannitol is an inert alcohol which does not readily penetrate animal epithelia. When the sodium chloride concentration in the perfusate was 65 mEq l^{-1}, or higher, fluid moved out of the proximal tubule lumen. When the perfusate sodium chloride concentration was less than 65 mEq l^{-1}, water moved into the tubule. Furthermore, the perfusate remained isosmotic with the plasma, even though there was a sodium chloride concentration gradient across the tubule epithelium of up to 35 mEq l^{-1}. Thus sodium moved against its concentration gradient and water did not. These experiments provided still further evidence that fluid reabsorption from the proximal tubule is an active process, possibly due to active sodium transport.[237]

There was still the possibility that sodium moved out of the tubule down an electrical gradient. This implies an area of negativity outside the tubule lumen towards which the positively-charged sodium ion would move passively. Water would then tend to follow the sodium in order to maintain osmotic equilibrium. Giebisch[58] had previously measured an average electrical potential difference of 20 millivolts (lumen negative) across the proximal tubule of *Necturus* during free-flow conditions. Whittembury[228] confirmed that an electrical potential difference identical in magnitude and sign exists during stopped-flow microperfusion. In the absence of measurable osmotic concentration or electrical gradients favourable to passive movement of fluid out of the proximal tubule of *Necturus*, it had to be assumed that fluid reabsorption is active. Furthermore, it is likely that water reabsorption is driven by active transport of sodium since the movement of water and sodium were proportional.

Studies on the mammalian nephron (primarily the rat) following research protocols very similar to those used in studies of *Necturus* have yielded similar results; that is, that water reabsorption in the proximal tubule of mammals depends upon sodium reabsorption.[61] Furthermore, they have helped to elucidate some of the mechanisms which may be responsible for water and solute movement in the nephron distal to the proximal tubule.

Micropuncture studies have been made on rats which were made diuretic by perfusing mannitol solutions into the jugular vein. During mannitol diuresis in the rat (Fig. 10), there is a depression of the reabsorption of water. Unlike the situation in non-diuretic animals, the sodium concentration in the proximal tubule fluid fell to levels some 30 to 50 mEq l^{-1} less than in the plasma. Fluid reabsorption continued (although at a depressed rate) and the tubule-fluid sodium concentration fell significantly. This suggested that the reabsorbed fluid is isosmotic to the plasma.

The principal effect of mannitol diuresis on the rat distal tubule and loop of Henle is to intensify the reabsorption of sodium. As indicated in Fig. 10, during osmotic (mannitol) diuresis, low sodium concentrations are established very early in the distal tubule. In non-diuretic rats, the early distal tubule sodium concentration is only slightly less than the plasma sodium concentration. This probably indicates that sodium reabsorption in the loop of Henle is even more intensified when a non-reabsorbable solute is in the tubule fluid.

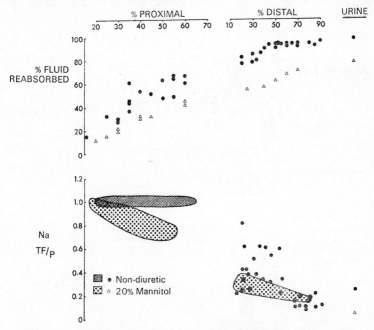

FIG. 10.   Sodium concentration and fluid reabsorption in the proximal and distal tubules of normal and diuretic (mannitol diuresis) rats. *Normal*: The sodium concentrations in the proximal tubule remain isomolar to the plasma and fall distally. *Diuretic*: The sodium concentration falls below that of the plasma in the proximal tubule and the hypomolarity is intensified distally. Fluid reabsorption in the proximal and distal tubules is 20–30% less than normal. From Giebisch and Windhager.[60]

Perfusion of albumen solutions into rat nephrons had effects identical to those seen in *Necturus*. In the rat, also, there was a reversal of flow of fluid into the tubule lumen after the experiment had progressed for some time. This was interpreted as being the consequence of the concentration of the lumenal fluid.[60]

Figure 11 illustrates the average transtubular electrical potentials which have been measured in various segments of the mammalian (rat and hamster) nephron.* It can be seen that in all segments sodium transport is against the electrical gradient. Even when the electrical potential is abolished by the short-circuiting technique, there is still a current measurable in both the amphibian (*Necturus*[47]) and mammalian (rat[236]) nephrons. The short-circuit technique consists of abolishing the transepithelial potential by applying an equal and opposite potential. When this is done, a flow of current may still be measurable. This current is

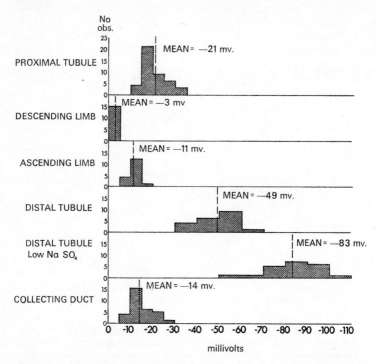

FIG. 11. Electrical potential differences in parts of the nephrons of hamsters (Henle's loop) and rats. When a non-reabsorbed anion ($SO_4^=$) is placed in the distal tubule of the rat, the transtubular potential rises sharply. From Giebisch and Windhager.[60]

---

* There is now reason to doubt that an electrical potential difference exists across the proximal tubule epithelium. In measurements made by Frömter and Hegel[55], the electrode tips were placed in the lumen and small amounts of fluid expelled, ascertaining that the electrodes were making contact with the tubule fluid. Under these conditions, no electrical potential differences were measured, even though prior to expelling fluid from the electrode, potential differences up to −80 millivolts were measured. It was confirmed that a potential difference averaging −60 millivolts exists across the distal tubule epithelium.

called the short-circuit current. Presumably it is related to the movement of charged particles by a mechanism other than the electrical potential difference.

Part of the fluid which leaves the lumen of the proximal tubule is attracted by colloids in the peritubular plasma. Laboratory rats have been injected subcutaneously with potassium dichromate, which causes necrosis (death) of the cells of the first two-thirds of the proximal tubule. The final urine of treated animals contained more glucose and protein, and it was more dilute than normal. Micropuncture studies of the damaged parts revealed that there was an abnormally rapid flow of fluid in the lumen; much less time was required to collect samples than is usual. The TF/P for inulin in the first and second thirds of the proximal tubule averaged 1·2 and 1·5 (normal inulin TF/P = 1·9 and 2·6, respectively). Since the tubule fluid was isosmotic to the general plasma, solutes were reabsorbed with water. It was possible that the measured inulin TF/P underestimated water reabsorption. The proximal tubule epithelium of dichromate-treated rats consisted of little more than a basement membrane. Inulin could easily have leaked out of the lumen.[64]

The filtration fraction of inulin bears an inverse relationship to the rate of fluid reabsorption from proximal tubules of rats. That is, the more fluid which enters the lumen of the proximal tubule, the faster is the rate of reabsorption. These results suggest that the oncotic pressure of colloids in the peritubular capillaries is responsible for a surprisingly large part of fluid reabsorbed from the proximal tubule.[100] The greater the proportion of fluid filtered from the plasma by the glomerulus, the greater would be the concentration of colloid in the plasma remaining. Since the remaining plasma passes directly to the peritubular capillaries, the colloid would tend to attract fluid from the proximal tubule lumen in proportion to its concentration.

Direct evidence for the foregoing proposition was provided by Spitzer and Windhager.[202] The lumena of proximal tubules of rat nephrons were blocked with an oil droplet and timed collections of fluid were made. The glomerular filtration rate could be calculated from a knowledge of the rate of fluid collection (= fluid flow) and the tubular fluid : plasma ratios for inulin. The difference between the GFR and the rate of fluid collection at the puncture site was the rate of fluid reabsorption between the glomerulus and the micropuncture site. The rate of fluid reabsorption from the lumen was determined first whilst the proximal tubules were perfused with plasma in the peritubular capillaries (controls, Table 3). The peritubular capillaries were then punctured with a second pipette (Fig. 12). The rate of fluid reabsorption was determined whilst the peritubular capillaries were perfused with

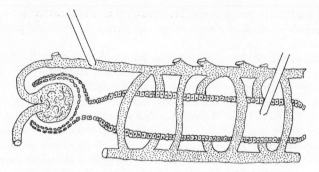

FIG. 12.   Method of collecting fluid from proximal tubules of animals whilst the peritubular capillaries are being perfused simultaneously with artificial solutions. From Spitzer and Windhager.[202]

Ringer or with Ringer containing 8 gm per 100 ml of dextran to simulate plasma colloid (experimentals). The results of these experiments (Table 3) showed clearly that fluid reabsorption from the proximal tubule lumen was reduced to about one-half normal when colloid-free Ringer was perfused through the peritubular capillaries.

Even under control conditions (Table 3), the fluid reabsorption rate seemed highly variable. Therefore, further experiments were

TABLE 3

Upper Table: reabsorption of normal tubule fluid during perfusion of the perfusion of the peritubular capillaries with blood (control), Ringer or Ringer containing 8% Dextran 110*. Values are given as mean plus or minus the standard error of the mean. Lower Table: reabsorptive capacity of the proximal tubules for saline droplets placed, in the lumen whilst the peritubular capillaries were perfused with blood (control) Ringer, and 4% and 8% Dextran 110 in Ringer. Values given as mean plus or minus the standard error of the mean. The statistical significance of the differences between the means of control and experimental data is given. Data from Spitzer and Windhager.[202]

	CAPILLARY PERFUSION FLUID			
	Ringer		8% Dextran	
	Control	Experimental	Control	Experimental
Reabsorption Rate ($nl\,min^{-1}$)	13.4 ± 2.1	6.4 ± 1.2	7.8 ± 1.1	8.7 ± 1.3
Significance		very significant		not significant

| | Control | Ringer | 4% Dextran | 8% Dextran |
| Reabsorption Capacity ($nl\,sec^{-1}\,mm$ surface) | 0.063 ± 0.003 | 0.031 ± 0.002 | 0.046 ± 0.004 | 0.060 ± 0.005 |

*Dextran 110 has an average molecular weight of 110 000 .

performed in which the load (amount) of fluid presented to the tubule epithelium did not vary. Accordingly, the split-droplet microperfusion technique (Fig. 4) was utilized to determine the rate of fluid reabsorption under constant load conditions. Droplets of Ringer were placed in the proximal tubule lumen. The peritubular capillaries were either unperfused (controls) or perfused with Ringer alone or Ringer containing 4% or 8% dextran. The rate of fluid reabsorption and the area of the tubule surface exposed to the perfusion-fluid droplets were measured. From these measurements the reabsorptive capacity, C, (i.e. the rate of fluid reabsorption relative to the area of tubule surface) could be calculated. The results, summarized in the lower part of Table 3, indicate clearly that when the peritubular capillaries are perfused with a colloid-free solution the reabsorptive capacity of the tubular epithelium is reduced by about one-half, but it is not abolished. Therefore, active metabolism of the cells and passive reabsorption due to plasma colloids contribute importantly to fluid reabsorption in the proximal tubule.

Chloride

There is no conclusive evidence that chloride is reabsorbed in the proximal tubule. In the mammal (rat[102]) and *Necturus* (Fig. 9), tubule fluid chloride concentration may exceed the chloride concentration of the plasma. It has been assumed that the electrochemical gradient across the proximal tubule is sufficient to cause chloride to leave the lumen passively. (In effect, the lumen is negative and chloride is more concentrated there; both factors should tend to force the negatively-charged chloride ion out of the lumen.) However, there must be some mechanism which opposes the movement of chloride out of the lumen. What this might be is purely a matter for speculation. Acidification of the urine occurs in the proximal tubule of the mammal. The rise in the chloride concentration can be correlated with the acidification.[59]

The large electrochemical gradient favours the movement of chloride from the distal tubule lumen, suggesting that chloride reabsorption there is passive. Finally, in the collecting ducts, there is good evidence that both sodium and chloride are actively reabsorbed.[78]

Sodium

Reabsorption of sodium from the tubule fluid in all parts of the amphibian nephron, and all parts of the mammalian nephron except the descending thin limb of Henle's loops, appears to be active. The energy for active sodium transport may be derived from aerobic metabolism. Several investigators have found that there is a linear relationship between oxygen consumption and sodium reasorptbion in the kidney.[60]

Therefore, it is rather puzzling that the kidney does not utilize oxygen to the same extent as do other tissues. The oxygen concentration of blood in the renal vein is about 80–90 per cent. of the oxygen concentration of blood in the renal artery. This compares with values of 50–70 per cent. in other tissues.[41] These two observations may be rationalized if it is assumed that sodium transport is very efficient; it has been calculated that the efficiency of the sodium transport in the mammalian kidney may be as high as 75%.[211]

In vertebrates in general, sodium chloride loading leads to retention of water in the tubule lumen with a concomitant diuresis. Two features

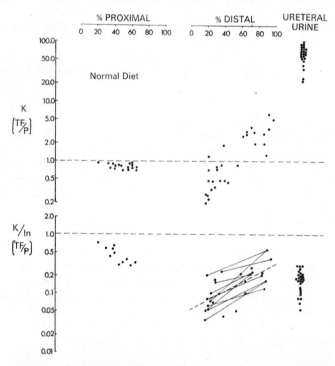

FIG. 13.   Tubule fluid : plasma and clearance ratios for potassium and inulin in various parts of the nephrons of rats maintained on a diet containing potassium. *Upper figure*: Potassium concentration in the proximal tubule is just hypomolar to the plasma. It appears to fall in the early distal tubule and rise in the late distal tubule. *Lower figure*: Clearance ratio $(K\ TF/P \div \text{inulin}\ TF/P)$ indicates that there is a net reabsorption of potassium in all parts of the nephron, although potassium is secreted in the distal tubule (dashed line, lower figure). From Giebisch and Windhager.[60]

of sodium excretion (at least in the laboratory rat) are not understood. First, only about 80% of the sodium chloride in the proximal tubule is available for reabsorption. Secondly, despite wide variations in the amounts of sodium entering the nephron, only about 75 to 80 per cent. is reabsorbed. Sodium reabsorption (and concomitant fluid reabsorption) therefore appears to be load-dependent. For a review of current hypotheses regarding this phenomenon, see references 60, 100A and 235.

Potassium

Potassium is one of the most variable constituents in urine; the potassium concentration of the final urine may exceed that of the plasma. Nevertheless, potassium : inulin clearance ratios indicate that less potassium is excreted than is filtered (Fig. 13). Clearance and stop-flow studies both indicate that most of the potassium which enters the proximal tubule is reabsorbed. Figure 14 illustrates the results of stop-flow studies of potassium excretion during mannitol diuresis. The concentration of potassium in the early urine samples (taken after flow is resumed) is high, indicating that the potassium concentration of the tubular fluid is augmented distally. The potassium : inulin clearance ratios are still less than unity in the final urine, indicating that potassium reabsorption has occurred.

Berliner,[9] and Berliner, Kennedy and Orloff[10] have postulated the existence of potassium : sodium and sodium : hydrogen ion exchange mechanisms in the distal tubule. These postulates arose primarily from two observations. First, urinary acidity bears an inverse relationship to sodium excretion; the higher the hydrogen ion concentration (i.e. lower the pH) of the urine, the lower the sodium concentration. Secondly, there is a direct relationship between the acidity of the urine and urinary potassium concentration.

Berliner[9] has developed the thesis that the bulk of the potassium in the final urine is derived from secretory processes in the distal tubule; this is a view based primarily on clearance studies of the ion. However, support for the hypothesis comes from some direct (micropuncture) studies. The potassium : inulin TF/P ratios (Fig. 13) fall in the proximal tubule and rise distally.[117] Comparison of the potassium present in the distal tubule with that in the final urine indicates that a minimum of about three-quarters of the potassium in the final urine is derived from the distal tubule.[60]

The electrical gradient and potassium reabsorption

Electrophysiological studies support the view that potassium entry into the distal tubule is determined by the transtubular electrical

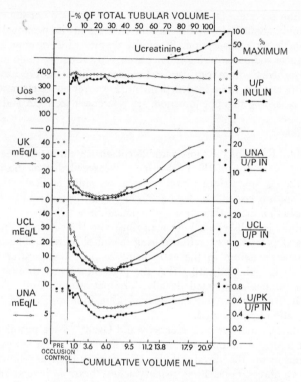

FIG. 14. Stop-flow studies or urine osmotic pressures, urine : plasma ratios of inulin, sodium, chloride and potassium, and clearance ratios for sodium, chloride and potassium. Sodium, chloride, potassium and water were reabsorbed distally whilst flow was stopped (occlusion). Reabsorption of sodium and chloride was especially marked during stoppage of flow. Resumption of flow (creatinine graph) caused the re-establishment of normal urine osmotic pressures and ion concentrations. From Jaenike and Berliner.[84]

gradient, not a sodium : potassium exchange mechanism.[60] The transtubular electrical potential difference may be increased by depositing a droplet of sodium chloride or sodium sulfate in the tubule lumen (Fig. 11). Under these conditions entry of potassium into the tubule is increased. If choline chloride (a substance which does not penetrate the epithelium) is placed in the distal tubule, the transtubular potential is virtually abolished. (This is seen also in the proximal tubule of *Necturus*.[228]) When the transtubular potential is virtually eliminated by choline, potassium entry into the lumen is greatly depressed. The placement of choline chloride into the lumen is followed also by the entry of large amounts of sodium. Therefore, lack of sodium for exchange could not explain the failure of potassium entry into the lumen.

Giebisch and Windhager[60] conclude from their review of the subject that it is unnecessary to postulate a carrier-linked potassium : sodium exchange in the distal tubule. The electrical potential across the tubular epithelium is sufficient to account for potassium movement into the lumen. However, there may be an electrical 'coupling' between transtubular sodium and potassium movement. That is, as potassium enters the lumen passively, it would enhance the exit of sodium by lowering the transtubular potential fractionally.

Calcium and magnesium

During saline diuresis, the amount of calcium and magnesium filtered (filtration fraction) appeared to fall; nevertheless, this led to the increased excretion of those two ions. Saline diuresis diminished sodium reabsorption, but its depressive effect on reabsorption of calcium and magnesium was more pronounced. This suggested that sodium, calcium and magnesium compete for common reabsorption sites on the mammalian nephron.[128] The presence of calcium in fluid perfused by the split-droplet method (Fig. 4) into the proximal tubule slows the rate of fluid reabsorption. This could be due to sodium : calcium competition for a common absorption site, but also it could indicate that calcium acts as a poorly reabsorbed ion in the manner of sulphate.[56]

Monosaccharides

Glucose disappears from the lumenal fluid within the proximal tubule of *Necturus*;[171] this is true also of the mammal.[220] The normal plasma glucose concentration in mammals is about 100 mg per 100 ml. A plasma glucose concentration in excess of *c.* 120 mg per 100 ml (in man) is known as hyperglycaemia, which may lead to the appearance of glucose in the final urine (glycosuria)[81]. Glycosuria can be induced also by the injection or infusion of the glycoside, phlorizin, into the blood.

The fact that hyperglycaemia and phlorizin poisoning cause glycosuria lends support to the view that reabsorption of glucose is an active process. Thus elevation of the plasma glucose increases the concentration of glucose in the proximal tubule fluid to a level where the transport (reabsorptive) mechanism becomes saturated. Phlorizin 'competes' with glucose for a carrier-binding site in the proximal tubule which has a greater affinity for phlorizin than for glucose.

c

Secretion in the nephron tubule

Organic acids and bases

Vertebrate kidneys secrete a very large variety of organic substances. Some appear to enter the urine via pathways which have narrowly-limited affinities. Perhaps only one or a few structurally similar compounds are handled by each such pathway. On the other hand, some secretory pathways handle a large number of compounds which are not necessarily structurally closely related. Throughout the vertebrates are recognized two of these generalized pathways, which appear to be confined to the proximal tubule. The first is responsible primarily for secreting organic acids; the second secretes organic bases. Common examples of compounds secreted by the organic acid pathway are diodrast (3,5-*di*-iodo-4-pyridone-N-acetic acid), *para*-amino hippuric acid (PAH), phenol red (phenolsulfonephthalein or PSP), and phlorizin. Some compounds secreted by the organic base pathway are tetraethylammonium (TEA), choline and 5-hydroxytryptamine (5-HT, serotonin). Two organic bases, creatinine and urea, appear to be secreted by the organic acid pathway. A curious feature of the organic acid and base secretory pathways is that they do not handle the same compounds uniformly in all vertebrates. Phenol red and PAH appear to be secreted uniformly, (except in hagfish, see below). Urea appears to be secreted by the frog but not by *Necturus* or mammals (Fig. 9). Further, creatinine appears to be secreted by *Necturus*, but not by some mammals (e.g. dog, see below) where it may be used to measure the glomerular filtration rate.

The organic acid and base secreting mechanisms exhibit the phenomena of secretory maxima and competitive inhibition. As shown in Fig. 15a, as the plasma concentration of phenol red is elevated, its secretion rate reaches a maximum. (However, the amount of phenol red excreted continues to increase, indicating that it is simultaneously filtered.) In Fig. 15b, the competitive effect of PAH and Diodrast is shown. When PAH is in the plasma alone, it is secreted rapidly (c. 25 μmole kg^{-1} hr^{-1}). Diodrast alone is secreted at a reduced rate (c. 5 μmole kg^{-1} hr^{-1}). When PAH and Diodrast are present together in equimolar concentration, the secretion rate of PAH is much reduced, whilst the secretion rate of Diodrast is little affected.[52]

The organic acid and base secretory mechanisms are both halted by inhibitors of cellular oxidation, such as cyanide. However, only the organic acid secreting mechanism is inhibited by Krebs cycle inhibitors such as malonate (Table 1). The organic base secreting mechanism is unaffected by such inhibitors.

The organic acid (PAH) secreting mechanism probably plays an

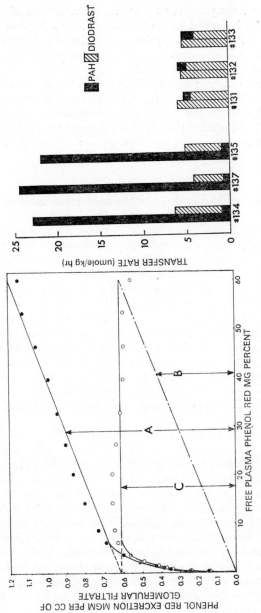

FIG. 15. *Left:* Excretion of phenol red in the chicken. Curve A shows the total excretion of phenol red, curve B the amount filtered. Curve C is the difference between the amount excreted and the amount filtered, which is the amount secreted. The amount secreted (C) rises to a maximum despite a rise in the plasma concentration; therefore a transport maximum is reached. From Pitts.[150] *Right:* The secretion of *para*-amino hippuric acid (PAH) and Diodrast by the aglomerular fish, *Lophius*. On the left are shown the rates of secretion of the two compounds individually. On the right are shown the effects of competitive inhibition when the two compounds are present in equimolar concentration. From Forster and Hong.[52]

important role in secreting unwanted products of metabolism. *Para-amino hippuric acid* is formed in the kidney by the conjugation of benzoic acid with the amino acid, glycine. By similar steps involving sulphuric and glucuronic acids, toxic materials may be excreted which otherwise could not penetrate the tubule.[199]

The mesonephric kidney of the hagfish, *Myxine* is unable to secrete phenol red, but the dye is secreted in the bile. This result is somewhat surprising. The tubule of the mesonephric kidney in *Myxine* is considered to be homologous to the proximal tubule of jawed vertebrates (Chapter 1), in which the ability to secrete phenol red appears to be uniform.

Monosaccharides

Recent studies have provided evidence of the mechanism involved in the uptake of glucose (dextrorotatory or '*D*' glucose) and a variety of other monosaccharides by kidney cells.[193,194] These studies may help clarify the process of secretion, although they provide no direct evidence that monosaccharides may be secreted. Silverman and his colleagues have utilized an elegant method called by the rather formidable name, the 'sudden-injection-multiple-indicator-dilution' technique to study the excretion of monosaccharides by the dog kidney. Changes in the concentrations of creatinine, T–1824 (Evans blue dye) and mono-saccharides in the renal vein were measured during a few minutes after injection of those compounds into the renal artery. Changes in the concentration of creatinine and monosaccharide in the urine were measured also. Because it is filtered by the dog kidney, creatinine may be utilized to measure extracellular volume in the kidney. Evans blue dye becomes bound to plasma proteins and is used to measure circulating blood volume.

The rationale of the experimental protocol of Silverman and his colleagues was as follows: a substance injected into the renal artery will be confined to the extracellular space if curves describing changes in the concentration of that substance in the renal vein and urine exactly overlap the curve for creatinine injected at the same time. Figure 16a shows such a curve for *L*-glucose, the form of glucose which is not reabsorbed by the vertebrate nephron. If the substance injected with creatinine and Evan's blue enters the cells of the nephron tubules, changes in the concentration of the substance in the renal vein blood and urine will be at variance with changes in the creatinine concentration. This can be illustrated with *D*-glucose, which is reabsorbed by the proximal tubule. When *D*-glucose is injected with creatinine into the renal artery, a fraction of the injected quantity will be filtered at the glomerulus. The amount remaining in the plasma will pass via the

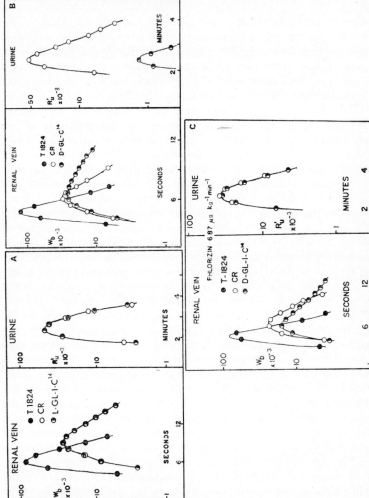

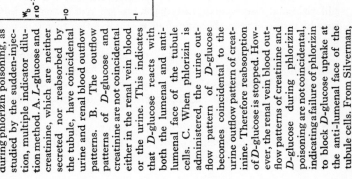

FIG. 16. Reaction of the proximal tubule to *L*-glucose and *D*-glucose during phlorizin poisoning, as studied by the sudden-injection, multiple indicator dilution method. A. *L*-glucose and creatinine, which are neither secreted nor reabsorbed by the tubule, have coincidental urine and renal blood outflow patterns. B. The outflow patterns of *D*-glucose and creatinine are not coincidental either in the renal vein blood or the urine. This indicates that *D*-glucose reacts with both the lumenal and anti-lumenal face of the tubule cells. C. When phlorizin is administered, the urine outflow pattern of *D*-glucose becomes coincidental to the urine outflow pattern of creatinine. Therefore reabsorption of *D*-glucose is stopped. However, the renal vein blood outflow patterns of creatinine and *D*-glucose during phlorizin poisoning are not coincidental, indicating a failure of phlorizin to block *D*-glucose uptake at the anti-lumenal face of the tubule cells. From Silverman, Aganon, and Chinard.[193]

efferent arteriole into the post-glomerular circulation. Most of the filtered glucose will be reabsorbed by the proximal tubule and passed into the peritubular capillaries. If creatinine and D-glucose occupy the same volume in the post-glomerular circulation, then it may be predicted that the concentration of D-glucose in the renal vein will equal or exceed the concentration of creatinine; the concentration of D-glucose will be augmented by an amount being reabsorbed by the tubules. However, if the concentration of glucose in the renal vein at any sampling period is less than the concentration of creatinine, then it may be predicted that D-glucose undergoes some kind of time-consuming interaction with the kidney tissue during passage through the post-glomerular circulation. As shown in Fig. 16b, the concentrations of D-glucose in the renal vein fall below those of creatinine. This result was thought to indicate that D-glucose becomes bound to or penetrates through the antilumenal surface of the nephron. The interaction of D-glucose with the antilumenal surface of the nephron could be demonstrated readily when lumenal glucose uptake was blocked with phlorizin. If there is no interaction between the antilumenal surface of the tubule and glucose, the concentrations of D-glucose and creatinine in the renal vein should coincide, as illustrated in Fig. 16a for L-glucose. Fig. 16c shows that phlorizin causes coincidence of the concentration curves for D-glucose and creatinine in the urine. However, D-glucose still occupies a greater space in the post-glomerular circulation than does creatinine; these results provided strong support for the contention that D-glucose is taken up or bound to the antilumenal surface of the tubule. One further interesting result can be inferred from Fig. 16c. Phlorizin does not block the binding or uptake of D-glucose at the antilumenal face of the nephron tubule at the same concentration as it takes to block uptake at the lumenal face. Further work showed that phlorizin must be present in a concentration about 1000 times that shown in Fig. 16c before it will inhibit binding or uptake of D-glucose at the antilumenal face. Silverman and his colleagues[193] concluded that the phlorizin and D-glucose uptake pathways are not common, but they may be very close together on the membrane so that they interfere with each other.

In further studies, Silverman and his colleagues[194] utilized the sudden-injection multiple-indicator dilution technique to study the structural characteristics of monosaccharides which make them susceptible to cellular uptake. Fourteen monosaccharides were studied. Table 4 shows the site of interaction (if any) with the tubule epithelium. The investigators come to the following conclusions. First, at the lumenal membrane of the proximal tubule there are two sets of sites for reabsorption of monosaccharides. At one set D-glucose,

TABLE 4

Interactions between the lumenal and antilumenal surfaces of the nephrons of the dog kidney and various monosaccharides. From Silverman, Aganon and Chinard.[194]

Monosaccharide	Lumenal	Antilumenal
D-glucose	yes	yes
2-deoxy-D-glucose	yes	no
3-O-methyl-D-glucose	no	yes
D-galactose	yes	yes
D-mannose	yes	yes
6-deoxy-D-galactose (D-fucose)	no	yes
D-xylose	no	yes
D-ribose	no	no
2-deoxy-D-ribose	no	no
L-glucose	no	no
L-arabinose	no	yes
6-deoxy-L-galactose (L-fucose)	no	no
D-arabinose	no	no
D-talose	no	yes

2-deoxy-*D*-glucose and *D*-galactose are reabsorbed, but the reabsorptive mechanism has varying affinities for the three monosaccharides. At the second set of sites *D*-mannose is reabsorbed. Secondly, for an interaction to take place at the lumenal and/or antilumenal membrane the reabsorbed monosaccharide must have a specific structural configuration. Important to this structural configuration is the existence of hydroxyl groups on specific carbon atoms, suggesting that the sugar : membrane interaction is due to hydrogen bonding. This would produce interactions of low average energy which could be disrupted easily.

Inorganic ions

As discussed in an earlier section, there is evidence that two ions, hydrogen and potassium, are secreted by the nephron of vertebrates.

Chapter 6

Concentration of the urine; an introduction

In all terrestrial vertebrates the urine may become concentrated due to water withdrawal. In the nephrons of reptiles and birds which lack Henle's loops, the greater amount of the water withdrawal appears to take place in the cloaca. As indicated by inulin urine : plasma ratios greater than unity, water is withdrawn from the urine of aquatic vertebrates; the final urine normally is more dilute than the plasma (freshwater vertebrates, marine teleosts) or isosmotic with the plasma (elasmobranchs). The hagfish, *Eptatretus stouti*[133] and *Myxine*,[158] are exceptional; apparently they do not withdraw water from their urine, since the inulin U/P is approximately unity.

In mammals and in the birds whose nephrons possess Henle's loops, water withdrawal from the urine occurs in the kidney, due to the highly organized arrangement of medullary and cortical components (Fig. 3). The urine-concentrating abilities of mammals are in general related to the size and extent of the medullary region of the kidney (Table 5). This, in turn, is related to the length of the thin segments of

TABLE 5

Relationship between thickness of the renal medulla, length of the nephrons and ability to concentrate the urine. Modified from Schmidt-Nielsen and O'Dell.[190]

Mammal	Percent long-looped nephrons	Relative medullary thickness	Max. urine freezing-point depression (°C)
Beaver	0	1·3	0·96
Pig	3	1·6	2·00
Man	14	3·0	2·60
Dog	100	4·3	4·85
Cat	100	4·8	5·8
Rat	28	5·8	4·85
Kangaroo Rat (*Dipodomys*)	27	8·5	10·4
Jerboa	33	9·3	12.0
Sand Rat (*Psammomys*)	100	10·7	9·2

the loops of Henle. The medullary region of the kidney in birds also takes part in the concentration of the urine.[195] However, the ability of birds to withdraw water from the urine appears to be related to the numbers of long-looped nephrons, rather than the length of the thin limbs of Henle's loops.[156]

Wirz, Hargitay and Kuhn[238] published experimental evidence that the counter-current principle may be utilized by mammals to withdraw water from the urine. Slices of tissue were taken from various levels of the renal medulla and the osmotic pressure was determined. In antidiuretic animals there was shown to be an increasing osmotic gradient from the outer medulla toward the renal papilla. It was suggested that this 'cortico-medullary' osmotic gradient is due to the countercurrent withdrawal of water in the medulla.

The operation of a countercurrent concentrating mechanism is illustrated in Fig. 17. The flow of fluid in the ascending limb of Henle's loop (AL) is counter to the flow of fluid in the descending limb (DL) and collecting duct (CD). It was suggested that solute (NaCl) is transported out of the ascending limb without a concomitant movement of water, establishing an osmotic gradient within the medullary interstitium. The gradient attracts water out of the adjacent descending limbs of Henle's loops and collecting ducts. Since the fluid in the collecting ducts leaves the medulla, there can be little further alteration in its concentration. The shading in Fig. 17 indicates that the concentrating effect is multiplied along an axial gradient going from the outer medulla to the inner medulla. Maximum concentration of sodium is reached in the inner medulla,[190] and little further concentration occurs between that level and the papillary tip.

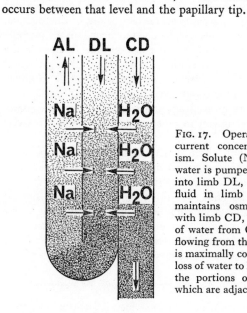

FIG. 17. Operation of a countercurrent concentration mechanism. Solute (Na) in excess of water is pumped out of limb AL into limb DL, concentrating the fluid in limb DL. Limb DL maintains osmotic equilibrium with limb CD, by the movement of water from CD to DL. Fluid flowing from the end of limb CD is maximally concentrated by the loss of water to limb DL all along the portions of the two limbs which are adjacent to each other.

There is no doubt that urine in mammals is concentrated because of the organization of the medulla. However, the significance of that organization is by no means clear. The countercurrent principle may be responsible for withdrawal of water from the medullary urine, but almost certainly not in the simple fashion illustrated in Fig. 17. All that could result would be a cycling of sodium between the ascending and descending limbs of Henle's loops. Some other mechanism would have to account for the removal of water from the medulla. In addition to the segments of the nephron, the renal medulla contains blood vessels, the vasa recta (Fig. 3) and a well-developed lymphatic system.[95,99] The elements of the circulatory system might function to remove water which leaves the nephron segments. A synthesis of the possible roles of both the nephric and circulatory elements in medullary urine concentration will be attempted after separate discussion of the possible roles of each element.

The role of medullary nephron segments in the concentration of the urine

Probably the primary difficulty encountered in studies of the mammalian concentrating mechanism is the inaccessibility of all parts of any single nephron. The cortical portions of some nephrons can be studied but these nephrons do not penetrate into accessible regions of the medulla. Conversely, portions of nephrons which penetrate deep into the medulla to the papilla can be studied, but their cortical portions lie deep in the inaccessible region of the cortex. Until some way is found to get round this difficulty, study of the concentrating mechanism must be relatively indirect. Conclusions drawn about events occurring in portions of nephrons not accessible to direct study must inevitably involve guess-work; they are therefore subject to more error than would otherwise be the case.

Within the medulla only three structures appear to be capable of performing osmotic work (i.e. actively maintaining an osmotic gradient); these are the ascending and descending limbs of Henle's loops and the collecting ducts. The vasa recta, like other capillaries, are considered to be incapable of producing an osmotic gradient across their walls. Studies of the possible mechanisms underlying concentration have tended to centre on the role of the ascending limb of Henle's loop, although the collecting duct is considered by some to play a part.

The Countercurrent hypothesis and the medullary nephron segments

The scheme of contercurrent concentration which is favoured generally involves the dilution of fluid in the ascending limb of Henle's loops relative to adjacent structures (Fig. 17). This dilution may be accom-

TABLE 6

Average tubule fluid: plasma ratios for osmolality, inulin and urea in various parts of the rat nephron. Also shown are clearance ratios for urea (Urea TF/P ÷ Inulin TF/P). From Davson[41] after Lassiter, Gottschalk and Mylle.

Source	Osmolality	Inulin	Urea	Urea clearance ratio
Early proximal	1·0	1·0	1·0	1·0
Late proximal	1·0	3·0	1·5	0·5
Early distal	0·7	6·9	7·7	1·1
Late distal	1·0	14·9	10·5	0·7
Ureteral urine	6·4	690	90	0·13

plished by pumping solute in excess of water out of the ascending limb. Evidence in support of this proposition arose from early micro-puncture studies. As shown in Table 6, fluid in the distal tubule of the rat has a lower osmotic pressure than does fluid in the late proximal tubule. Furthermore, the inulin TF/P in the early distal tubule is about two and one-half times the inulin TF/P in the late proximal tubule. Therefore, there is a net water withdrawal in the loops of Henle.[41]

The renal papilla of the hamster can be made accessible to micro-puncture by opening the renal pelvis. Analyses of micropuncture samples taken from the tip of the hamster renal papilla (Table 7) showed that with respect to all major solutes the fluid at the bend of

TABLE 7

Tubule fluid: plasma ratios of various parameters, measured at the tip of the urinary papilla of the hamster. From Gottschalk.[65]

Parameter	Loop of Henle fluid	Collecting duct fluid
Osmolality	2·8	3·0
Inulin	11	122
Sodium	1·9	0·3
Chloride	2·8	0·8
Urea	17	54
pH	7·34	6·58

the thin limbs of Henle's loops is highly concentrated relative to fluid in the late proximal tubule of the rat (Table 6). The foregoing studies seemed to confirm the correctness of the main outlines of the counter-current hypothesis. That is, the tubule fluid becomes concentrated in the descending limbs of Henle's loop and solute in excess of water is withdrawn from the tubule fluid between the bend of Henle's loop and the early part of the distal tubule.

The role of sodium in the urine-concentrating process. Mammals produce urine which has a low sodium concentration. Further, the fluid in the early distal tubule of mammals has a low sodium concen-tration. Therefore, the countercurrent mechanism may involve the active transport of sodium out of the ascending limb of Henle's loop without a concomitant movement of water. The rise in the sodium concentration of the medullary interstitium may cause the osmotic withdrawal of water from the descending limb of Henle's loop and the collecting duct. Water removal from the collecting ducts finally concen-trates the urine. This suggests that sodium may be cycled between the ascending and descending limbs of Henle's loops.

The role of urea in the urine-concentration process. Urea probably enters the tubule fluid in the Henle's loops, since its concentration in the early part of the distal tubule is over five times its concentration in the late proximal tubule (of the rat). Furthermore, comparison of the urea : inulin clearance ratios (Table 6) shows that urea is reabsorbed from all parts of the rat nephron except Henle's loops. In the hamster (Table 7) the concentration gradient for urea between the collecting duct and loops of Henle probably favours the backflow of urea out of the collecting ducts into the medullary interstitium. Like sodium, urea is probably cycled within the medulla of the kidney, but it is not clear whether or not this cycling process occurs between the limbs of Henle's loops or between the limbs of Henle's loops and the collecting duct. As shown by several studies[234] urea contributes significantly to maximal concentration of the urine in mammals.

Recent studies of the countercurrent mechanism

Many indirect studies support the view that the countercurrent principle is involved in the concentration of the urine of mammals (see Windhager, reference 234). Some direct studies[65] also support this view, but only in relation to the outer medulla where the thick portions of Henle's loops are located. Maximum medullary withdrawal of water from the urine occurs within the inner medulla where the thin segments of Henle's loops are found. Recent direct studies have been concerned with attempts to analyze the role of the thin limbs in the concentration of the urine.

The main features of the countercurrent concentrating mechanism will be summarized as a series of propositions, which will serve as a framework for discussion of recent studies of the concentration mechanism as it may operate in the inner medulla.

1. The source of osmotic work in the renal medulla is active transport of sodium out of the ascending thin limb of Henle's loops. The interstitium is thereby concentrated, attracting water from adjacent descending limbs, collecting ducts and blood vessels.
2. The ascending limb of Henle's loop is impermeable to water. Active transport of sodium out of the ascending limb tends to dilute the fluid in the lumen.
3. The descending limb of Henle's loop, the collecting ducts and capillaries of the vasa recta are passively permeable to water and small solute molecules.

1. *The ascending limb of Henle's loop is the source of osmotic work in the renal medulla.* Solute and water transport by the thin limbs of Henle's loops in the hamster has been studied using the stopped-flow microperfusion technique.[65,122] In one study (Gottschalk),[65] solute, but not water, was reabsorbed from ascending limbs and both solute and

water were reabsorbed from the descending lmbs. These findings appeared to confirm the major feature of the countercurrent hypothesis: the ascending thin limb of Henle's loop is capable of transporting solute in the absence of net water movement. However, in a second study (Marsh and Solomon)[122] in which the experimental protocol was almost identical to the first, the opposite result was obtained. That is, saline solutions perfused into the ascending and descending limbs of Henle's loops did not change composition and fluid was not reabsorbed. In the studies both of Gottschalk and of Marsh and Solomon, perfusion of the thin limbs with solutions containing the non-reabsorbable sugar, raffinose, caused fluid to move into the loops, showing that the loops are permeable to water.

Measurements of electrical potential differences across the walls of the ascending and descending thin limbs of Henle's loops, vasa recta and collecting ducts have been made by Windhager[233] and by Marsh and Solomon.[122] Under free-flow conditions in anti-diuretic animals, only very small potential differences could be measured across the descending limbs (Fig. 11) and vasa recta. Under similar conditions potential differences averaging -9 to -11 millivolts and -14 to -17 millivolts (lumen negative) were measured, respectively, across the ascending thin limbs and collecting ducts. During osmotic diuresis (free flow) or during stopped-flow microperfusion experiments the potential difference across the ascending thin limb was greatly diminished or abolished; the small potential difference across the descending limb was unaffected.

The existence of an electrical potential difference across the wall of the thin ascending Henle's loop would seem to support the thesis that solute is transported actively out of that segment. When the ascending limb is perfused continuously with concentrated saline, the free-flow electrical potential differences seen during antidiuresis (i.e. descending limb $= -3$ mV, ascending limb $= -11$ mV) persist. The potential differences could be abolished with metabolic inhibitors, suggesting that they are maintained by cellular metabolism.[233] In some unknown way, stopped-flow microperfusion may alter the permeability characteristics of the thin limbs so that they no longer function normally. The normal transepithelial electrical potential differences are abolished.

Evidence derived from direct study of the ascending thin limbs of Henle's loops does not provide unqualified support for the correctness of the first proposition. The ascending limb may be capable of osmotic work, but unequivocal evidence is still lacking.

2. *The ascending limb is impermeable to water; other medullary nephric and vascular elements are passively permeable to water and small*

solute molecules. Morgan and Berliner[132] studied the permeability of the loops of Henle, collecting ducts and vasa recta in isolated renal papillae of the laboratory rat. Prior to excision of the papillae, dilute solutions were infused into the rats, abolishing the medullary osmotic gradient. The papillae were isolated in isosmolal (500 mosmoles) or hyperosmolal (700 mosmoles) media. Antidiuretic hormone (ADH) was added to the medium in some experiments (see p. 72 below). The lumena of the isolated nephron segments and vasa recta were perfused with saline containing radioactive (tritiated) water, urea and inulin. The concentration of the perfusing saline was always 500 mosmoles. A perfusing pipette was placed in the lumen of the nephron tubule or vas rectum and timed collections made into a second pipette placed downstream from the first. The diameter and length of the perfused segment and changes in the concentrations of water, urea, inulin and sodium during perfusion were measured. The diffusional permeability (i.e. permeability in the absence of a concentration or hydrostatic gradient) of the various epithelia were calculated. Also calculated were the diffusional permeability to water and urea and the net fluxes of water, urea and solutes.

The diffusional permeabilities of the nephron segments and vasa recta to water and urea are summarized in Table 8. The diffusional permeability to water of the descending limb of Henle's loop is over

TABLE 8

Diffusive permeability of perfused medullary segments of rat nephrons and vasa recta to tritiated water (^3H_2O) and radioactive urea. The medullary segments were bathed in media in which anti-diuretic hormone (ADH) was present or absent, as indicated. The osmolalities of perfusion and bathing media were the same (500 milliosmoles). Values are expressed as the mean plus or minus the standard error of the mean. The mean values in bold-face type are very significantly different (statistically). From Morgan and Berliner.[132]

Perfused segment	^3H_2O permeability coefficient (cm sec$^{-1} \times 10^{-5}$)		^{14}C-urea permeability coefficient (cm sec$^{-1} \times 10^{-5}$)	
	no ADH	ADH	no ADH	ADH
Descending limb	119±14	95±10	13±3·0	20±4·3
Ascending limb	50±4·5	39±2·6	14±2·0	16±2·8
Collecting ducts	**45±3·1**	**87±7·4**	20±1·3	**30±2·4**
Vasa recta	192±20	201±25	47±3·3	66±6·0

twice that of the ascending limb and collecting duct. However, the three medullary nephron segments all have similar diffusional permeabilities to urea. Antidiuretic hormone increases the diffusional permeability of the collecting ducts, but it has no effect on the other medullary structures. In the absence of an osmotic gradient, passive permeability to water of the descending limb of Henle's loop and the vasa recta is high relative to the other medullary structures.

An osmotic gradient was imposed across the tubular segments and vasa recta. Isolated renal papillae were bathed in a medium whose concentration was 700 mosmoles (= saline plus 200 mosmoles mannitol). The tubular segments and vasa recta were then perfused with 500 milliosmolal saline. Under these conditions (Table 9) there was a net

TABLE 9

Net water flux (nl cm^{-2}min^{-1} per milliosmole of concentration difference) out of thin limbs of the loops of Henle, collecting ducts and vasa recta of rats. Renal papillae were isolated in a bathing medium containing saline plus 200 milliosmoles per litre of mannitol, to make a total osmotic concentration of 700 milliosmoles. The nephron segments and vasa recta were perfused with saline whose concentration was 500 milliosmoles. Values are given as mean plus or minus the standard error. Data from Morgan and Berliner.[132]

	Loop of Henle*		Collecting ducts		Vasa recta
	Descending	Ascending	no ADH	ADH	
Net water flux	58±6·2	4·4±1·1	4·2±2·2	30±2·2	41±6·6

*ADH had no effect.

outward water flux from the medullary components. The magnitude of the flux was least from ascending limbs of Henle's loops and collecting ducts. Here again, ADH increased the water permeability of the collecting ducts, but it had no effect on the other medullary components.

Bearing in mind that in the studies of Morgan and Berliner medullary tissues were subjected to highly artificial conditions, the results support the proposition that the ascending thin limb of Henle's loop is relatively impermeable to water. However, the results provide no support for the contention that sodium is transported actively out of the ascending thin limb.

The micropuncture technique has been utilized by Jamison and his colleagues[85,86] to study changes in the osmolality and the concentrations of inulin, sodium and potassium in the thin limbs of Henle's loops. Access to the renal papilla of laboratory rats was by excision of large parts of the kidney tissue, a procedure which diminishes the ability of the kidney to concentrate the urine. The results of these studies (Table 10, upper part) indicate that fluid in the ascending limb of Henle's loop has a lower osmolality and a higher inulin concentration than does fluid in the descending thin limb. This indicates that solute in excess of water is withdrawn from the ascending thin limb. Furthermore, it appears that sodium is withdrawn from the ascending limb. From these studies it was concluded that the ascending limb of Henle's loop is the source of

TABLE 10

Changes in osmolality, tubule fluid: plasma ratios of sodium, potassium and inulin, and the sodium and potassium clearance ratios in the loops of Henle in the rat kidney. Data are expressed as the mean plus or minus the standard error. The statistical significance of differences between the values of parameters between the descending and ascending thin limbs of Henle's loops is given. Data from Jamison, apart from TF/P inulin*, which are from Horster and Thurau.[79]

Parameter	Descending limb	Bend	Ascending limb	Descending minus ascending	Significance
Osmolality (mosmoles)	581 ± 25	550 ± 39	525 ± 12	56	significant
TF/P inulin	4.31 ± 0.22	4.45 ± 0.10	5.92 ± 0.45	-1.61	very significant
TF/P sodium	1.55 ± 0.04	1.43 ± 0.07	1.45 ± 0.04	0.10	not significant
TF/P potassium	2.76 ± 0.19	3.81 ± 0.45	3.82 ± 0.36	-1.06	very significant
TF/P Na ÷ TF/P inulin	0.37 ± 0.02	0.34 ± 0.03	0.27 ± 0.02	0.10	very significant
TF/P K ÷ TF/P inulin	0.65 ± 0.05	0.87 ± 0.07	0.69 ± 0.06	-0.04	not significant
TF/P inulin*	25.0 ± 5.2	10.2 ± 5.2	6.9 ± 4.0		

osmotic work in the rat renal medulla. The medullary osmotic gradient is established by active transport of sodium out of the ascending limb. Initially, at least, sodium is accompanied by water, but ultimately dilution of the ascending limb fluid results.[85]

Unfortunately, results reported by Horster and Thurau[79] are directly contradictory to the above (Table 10, lower part). The inulin TF/P diminishes between the descending and ascending thin limbs of Henle's loops, indicating that fluid enters the loops in the ascending limb. Why there should be such wide disparity between two studies done on the same animal using very similar experimental protocols is not clear, but the answer may be provided by studies of Marsh.[121] Marsh measured changes in the osmolality and concentrations of inulin, sodium, potassium and urea in paired collections from the ascending and descending thin limbs of the Henle's loops of the hamster. Samples from the ascending limb were collected as follows. An oil-filled micropipette was inserted into a loop of Henle at its bend. A droplet of oil was expressed and watched as it flowed up the ascending limb. A second micropipette was inserted in the lumen of the ascending limb of the same loop of Henle, as visualized by the moving oil droplet. Tubule fluid samples were taken into both pipettes. Samples from the descending thin limbs were taken by reversing the foregoing procedure.

The results of Marsh's study are summarized in Table 11. The fluid in Henle's loop becomes more dilute and loses sodium and potassium going from the bend up into the first millimetre or so of the ascending limb. There appears to be no movement of water into or out of the ascending limb. However, there was a marked influx of urea.

TABLE 11

Osmolality, inulin TF/P *and concentrations of sodium, potassium and urea of fluid in the ascending and descending thin limbs relative to those values in fluid at the bend of the thin limbs of Henle's loops in the hamster kidney. Osmolality, and sodium, potassium and urea concentrations relative to inulin concentrations in the ascending and descending thin limbs relative to the bend of the loops of Henle. Data are expressed as means plus or minus the standard error of the mean. Values in bold-face type indicate that the mean is statistically different from unity. Data from Marsh.[121]*

Parameter	Ascending limb/bend	Bend/descending limb
Inulin TF/P	1·03 ± 0·023	**1·09 ± 0·037**
Osmolality	**0·94 ± 0·009**	**1·10 ± 0·030**
Sodium	**0·86 ± 0·020**	**1·08 ± 0·024**
Potassium	**0·86 ± 0·030**	1·02 ± 0·065
Urea	**1·20 ± 0·058**	**1·57 ± 0·089**
Osmolality/Inulin	**0·93 ± 0·025**	1·00 ± 0·047
Na/Inulin	**0·84 ± 0·024**	1·01 ± 0·028
K/Inulin	**0·84 ± 0·035**	0·95 ± 0·053
Urea/Inulin	**1·16 ± 0·049**	**1·52**

In going down the last millimetre or so of the descending limb, water is lost from the lumen so that the tubule fluid becomes more concentrated. The tubule fluid also gains sodium and urea, but the potassium concentration does not change.

Marsh concluded that his results are compatible with the hypothesis that active transport of sodium out of the ascending limb of Henle's loop drives the concentrating mechanism. He also suggested that the discrepancy between the results of Jamison and his colleagues,[85,86] and Horster and Thurau[79] was due possibly to sampling technique. In both studies, and in fact, all previous studies of thin loops, samples were taken randomly from loops of Henle in different experimental animals. Since the concentration of the renal medulla is highly variable from animal to animal and even in the same animal at different times, random samples are inherently subject to greater error.

Marsh and his colleague Solomon,[122] it may be recalled, had earlier concluded that the ascending thin limbs of Henle's loops are incapable of performing osmotic work. Saline solutions perfused into ascending thin limbs of the loop of Henle in the hamster did not change in volume or concentration. Marsh discussed alternative reasons which would make the stopped-flow microperfusion studies compatible with his most recent micropuncture studies. Stopped-flow studies are technically more difficult than micropuncture studies; they are subject, therefore to greater error. Marsh concluded that the results of the earlier studies with Solomon were due to some unknown source of error, despite the fact that he was able to repeat them, with the same result.

All available evidence from micropuncture and stopped-flow microperfusion studies indicates that the ascending limb of Henle's loop must be the source of osmotic work in the renal medulla, even though there is still no direct proof of this.

In their study of the sand rat, *Psammomys*, de Rouffignac and Morel[185] came to conclusions similar to those of Marsh; namely, there is no large net movement of water into or out of the loops of Henle. Fluid in the descending limb becomes concentrated by the addition of solutes, namely sodium, potassium and urea. Furthermore, in the ascending limb, sodium and potassium are reabsorbed, but there is no dilution of the fluid. There was no evidence that urea is reabsorbed in the ascending limb; this was taken to indicate that the ascending limb is impermeable to urea. However, it could equally be taken to indicate the net addition of urea to the ascending limb fluid as found by Marsh to be true in the hamster.

In conclusion, micropuncture and related studies of the nephron segments in the renal medulla and the vasa recta indicate that the ascending limb of Henle's loop is the most probable site of osmotic work. The descending limb and vasa recta probably play a passive role. The collecting ducts are capable also of active sodium transport.[78,120] It was suggested earlier that the collecting ducts could be the source of osmotic work in the medulla by transporting a hyperosmotic fluid out of the collecting ducts.[120] However, this suggestion has been abandoned.[121]

3. *The vasa recta and renal lymphatics play a passive role in the urine-concentration processes.* The circulatory elements undoubtedly play an important part in urine concentration. Whereas nephron segments are probably responsible for establishing the osmotic gradients necessary to concentrate urine, the circulatory elements probably maintain these gradients.

Numerous studies indicate that during diuresis medullary blood flow increases markedly,[11,234] eliminating the cortico-medullary concentration gradient. Direct measurement of the osmolality of vasa recta plasma[86,121] indicates a general similarity with fluid in the thin limbs of Henle's loops. However, Jamison and his colleagues[86] noted that the osmolality of the plasma, as compared to the osmolality of fluid in Henle's loops, varies with the rate of flow in the vasa recta. When blood flow was normal, plasma in the descending vasa recta was hypoosmotic to fluid in the lumen of the descending thin limb of Henle's loop, and isosmotic to fluid in the ascending limb of Henle's loop. When blood flow was slow, the osmolality of plasma in the descending vasa recta was isosmotic to fluid in the descending thin limb of Henle's loop, and hyperosmotic to fluid in the ascending thin limb. These results suggested that osmotic equilibrium between the vasa recta and the thin limbs of Henle's loops depends upon the rate of flow in the vasa recta. An increase in the concentration of fluid in the thin limbs probably depends upon the entry of solute into the descending thin limbs. When flow in the vasa recta is rapid, equilibrium between the descending vasa recta and descending limbs of Henle's loops is delayed. The descending vasa recta drain areas of the kidney (outer medulla, Fig. 3 p. 7) where the osmotic concentration is low relative to the inner medulla. Therefore rapid flow and delayed equilibrium will have the effect of diluting the medullary regions, abolishing the cortico-medullary concentration gradient.

Le Brie and Mayerson[99] and Le Brie[98] have attempted to assess the role of the renal lymphatics in urine concentration. The lymphatics are tortuous passages which lie adjacent to the cells. Part of their function is to return fluid to the vascular system via large lymph ducts which empty into the veins. When saline, mannitol and urea solutions were infused into dogs, an osmotic diuresis was induced. However, collections of fluid from the renal lymphatics revealed that only mannitol and saline solutions increased lymph flow. The interpretation put on these results was that all three substances are filtered out of the capillaries. However, saline and mannitol are retained in the extracellular space whilst urea freely enters the cells and the nephron lumena. These results suggest that during osmotic diuresis there is increased water loss from the vasa recta. The increased water loss may be attributable to increased medullary plasma flow and/or a decrease in the oncotic pressure of the blood plasma, the decrease in oncotic pressure of the plasma being a concomittant of a decrease in the amount of water filtered through the glomerulus.[98]

In rats maintained on a high sodium diet, the *GFR* of juxtamedullary nephrons diminished appreciably (Table 2). Further, the contribution of the juxtamedullary glomeruli to the whole kidney *GFR* diminished to about 12 %, as compared to 42 % in rats maintained on a low sodium diet. Since the whole kidney *GFR* increased by about 9 % in animals maintained on a high sodium diet, there was a marginal diuresis. Even if it is assumed that the total blood flow to the medulla does not alter (and several studies indicate that it increases),[98] it appears likely that more of the fluid passing through the juxtamedullary glomeruli would be shunted into the post-glomerular circulation, thus into the vasa recta. This would have the effect of expanding the medullary extracellular water content and diminishing water reabsorption from the collecting ducts. At the same time, solute entry into the descending thin limb of Henle's loops would increase.

Figure 18 represents a summary of the contribution made by all of the medullary elements during antidiuresis (Fig. 18a) and osmotic diuresis (Fig. 18b). The arrangement of the vasa recta relative to the thin limbs of Henle's loops is based on the anatomical studies of the kidney of the rat. Kriz[92] has demonstrated that the vasa recta lie close to the descending limb of Henle's loops, whilst the ascending limb and the collecting duct lie close together. The arrangement of the lymphatics relative to the vasa recta is based on studies of Takeuchi and his colleagues,[206] who demonstrated that the lymphatics are adjacent to the vasa recta.

Figure 18a depicts events which may occur during antidiuresis. An elevated *GFR* in juxtamedullary nephrons causes the rate of flow to increase in the descending limb of Henle's loop and to diminish in the vasa recta. As a consequence, osmotic equilibrium between the vasa recta and the descending limb occurs. Solutes move from the interstitium into both the vasa recta and descending limb and water moves out into the interstitium. Deep in the medulla, the vasa recta plasma and descending limb fluid are greatly concentrated.

Sodium is transported actively out of the ascending limb of Henle's loop into the interstitium. The osmotic gradient between the ascending limb and interstitium diminishes as the cortex is approached due to osmotic withdrawal of water from the adjacent collecting ducts and descending vasa recta. Continual withdrawal of water in excess of sodium and urea from the collecting ducts concentrates the fluid there. However, active transport of sodium and (probably) passive movement of urea out of the collecting duct occurs so that the urine is meagre in quantity and has a low sodium content. The sodium withdrawn from the collecting ducts and ascending thin limb may remain in the medulla, by entering the descending limb, or it may leave the medulla via the ascending vasa recta and lymph vessels. The urea withdrawn from the collecting ducts enters both limbs of Henle's loop, and in the ascending limb the urea compensates in part for the diminution of osmotic pressure due to the loss of sodium.

Figure 18b illustrates conditions which may prevail in the medulla when the urine is not being concentrated (i.e. during osmotic diuresis). Diminished GFR in the juxtamedullary nephrons shunts a greater part of the plasma into the vasa recta. This increases the volume of plasma flow through the medulla and the rate of fluid loss from the capillaries. Rapid plasma flow in the descending vasa recta hinders the establishment of concentration gradients between the vasa and the medullary interstitium, preventing concentration. Fluid in the descending limb of Henle's loop becomes equilibrated with the surrounding interstitium. Active sodium transport from the ascending limb still proceeds, but this is not effective in concentrating the interstitium because rapid plasma and lymph flow carry away the solute. Water reabsorption from the collecting duct is greatly diminished due to the lack of a large osmotic gradient. Therefore, a copious urine nearly isosmotic with the blood plasma is produced.

During water diuresis, a copious urine is produced, but it may be more concentrated with respect to certain solutes such as sodium. The GFR of juxtamedullary nephrons may not increase to quite the same extent as in osmotic diuresis. Alternatively, there may be less solute tending to retain water in the tubule fluid. Therefore, a condition intermediate between the two illustrated in Fig. 18 may exist.

Undoubtedly Fig. 18 represents a gross simplification of events, but it seems likely that any such scheme will suffer from several weaknesses, due simply to lack of knowledge of many of the processes that are involved.

Although sodium and urea play an important role in the concentration of the urine, other solutes, such as amino acids and protein may also be essential. The concentration gradient for plasma albumen parallels the osmotic gradient during antidiuresis.[33] There is disagree-

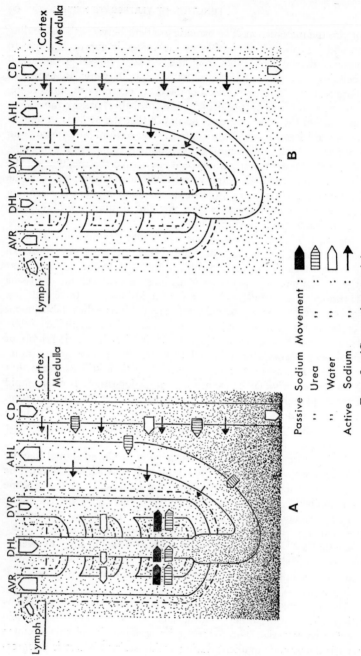

Passive Sodium Movement : ◄
" Urea " : ▯
" Water " : ▱
Active Sodium " : ↑

Fig. 18. (See caption opposite)

ment about the location of the albumen within the medulla. Some investigators believe that it is entirely vascular;[33] others consider at least part of the medullary albumen to be extravascular.[198]

Carone and his colleagues[33] believe that water may be filtered from the descending vasa recta by hydrostatic pressure, diminishing plasma flow in the medulla. Diminished plasma flow would then lead to the removal of water from the nephron tubule segments due to the oncotic pressure of plasma protein. Two major defects in this argument may be discerned: first, a hydrostatic pressure sufficient to effect filtration from the descending vasa recta does not appear to exist in the medulla during antidiuresis.[234] Furthermore, water would have to move out of the ascending limb of Henle's loops and recent micropuncture studies do not support this. It can be seen in Fig. 18 that a high rate of glomerular filtration in the juxtamedullary glomeruli will increase the oncotic pressure and diminish the rate of flow of plasma in the descending vasa recta. Therefore, the urine could be concentrated due to the oncotic uptake of water from the interstitium by colloids in the ascending vasa recta.

FIG. 18 (*opposite*).   Postulated events in the inner medulla of the mammalian kidney during anti-diuresis and osmotic diuresis. A. *Antidiuresis*: An increased glomerular filtration rate in the juxtamedullary nephrons shunts more of the medullary plasma into the descending limb of Henle's loop (DHL), slowing flow of plasma in the descending *vasa recta* (DVR), and diminishing flow in the lymphatic vessels (dashed lines). Active transport of solute (sodium) out of the ascending limb of Henle's loop (AHL) is now effective in concentrating the medullary interstitium; slowed plasma flow in the *vasa* and lymphatics allows a cortico-medullary osmotic gradient to be maintained. Urea moves passively into the ascending and descending limbs of Henle's loops and descending *vasa recta*, and out of the ascending *vasa recta*. Sodium moves passively into the descending *vasa recta* and descending Henle's loop, and out of the ascending *vasa recta*. Water moves passively out of the descending *vasa recta* and descending Henle's loop, and into the ascending *vasa recta*. Passive movements of sodium, urea and water adjust the osmotic equilibrium at all levels of the medulla, except within the ascending limb of Henle's loop and the collecting duct. Sodium is actively transported out of the collecting duct; water and probably urea move passively out of the collecting duct. The urine which leaves the medulla is concentrated, and it has a low sodium concentration. B. *Osmotic diuresis*: The GFR of juxtamedullary nephrons is diminished, shunting more of the medullary plasma into the descending *vasa recta*. Rapid flow of plasma which is isosmotic to the cortex in the descending *vasa recta* increases filtration into the lymphatics, preventing the accumulation of solute necessary for concentration. Active transport of sodium out of the ascending limb of Henle's loop and collecting duct is no longer effective in concentrating the interstitium. The high interstitial water content prevents reabsorption of water from the collecting duct and the urine produced is copious, but still isosmotic with the medulla.

Hormones and the mammalian kidney

The kidney is implicated as a site of action of several hormones which affect water and electrolyte balance. These include the steroid mineralo-corticoids produced by the adrenal cortex, the proteinaceous para-thyroid hormone and various peptide hormones of the neurohypophysis. The mineralocorticoids seem to effect an increased excretion of sodium, chloride and water. The hormone which is most closely implicated in these effects is 11-deoxycorticosterone, which appears to be involved with the sodium : hydrogen and sodium : potassium 'exchange' in the distal tubule. The parathyroid hormone appears to be implicated primarily in calcium and phosphate metabolism. It appears to bring about renal elimination of the ionic forms of those substances.

The hormones which have received most attention with respect to renal function are the octapeptide hormones of the posterior lobe of the pituitary (neurohypophysis). In mammals these are oxytocin and vasopressin (pitressin), whilst in non-mammals they are oxytocin and vasotocin. Oxytocin has marked effects on the contraction of smooth muscle. Its anti-diuretic action could be due to this. It could bring about contraction of the post-glomerular (efferent) arteriole, increasing the GFR and diminishing plasma flow through the vasa recta in the juxta-medullary glomeruli. The juxtamedullary glomeruli appear to lack the means of autoregulation of intraglomerular pressures (juxtaglomerular apparatus) possessed by cortical glomeruli.

The hormones whose actions on the kidney are best understood are the anti-diuretic hormones, arginine vasopressin in mammals and arginine vasotocin in non-mammals, particularly amphibians and fishes. For convenience these hormones will be designated ADH. The action of ADH has been reviewed by Leaf,[97] Orloff and Handler,[137] and Bentley.[7] The reader is referred to these for details.

Antidiuretic hormone acts primarily to increase the permeability of epithelia to water. In the kidney, this causes increased reabsorption of water from the distal tubule and collecting ducts. At the same time there may be an increase in the passive permeability of the epithelia to some solutes. In some tissues ADH may accelerate active transport of sodium. To be effective in isolated tissues the hormone must be placed in the side of the epithelium normally bathed by the blood. Antidiuretic hormone may act by mechanically or chemically altering the structure of epithelial membranes. However, recent evidence suggests that its main effect is exerted upon certain aspects of cellular metabolism.

There is good evidence that ADH becomes bound to receptor sites on cell membranes and in some way stimulates the intracellular production of the nucleotide, 3',5'-cyclic-adenosine monophosphate

(3',5'-cyclic AMP). However, the way in which cyclic AMP brings about a change in the permeability of the epithelium is unknown. In some tissues there appears to be an increase in sodium and potassium transport, suggesting that cyclic AMP stimulates pumps of some kind.

Appendix to part 2
Function of the aglomerular nephron

Smith,[199] Forster,[51] and Hickman and Trump[77] have summarized studies on aglomerular kidneys, and the reader is referred to those reviews for details and references.

The tubules of aglomerular nephrons have been considered to correspond to the proximal tubules in glomerular nephrons. This contention has received some support from ultrastructural studies[77] (Fig. 2). The aglomerular kidneys perform many of the same functions as do the proximal tubules of glomerular nephrons. They secrete a wide variety of compounds: phenol red, other dyes, creatinine, urea, uric acid and plasma ions. However, they presumably transport fluid in the opposite direction to the proximal tubules in glomerular nephrons. Inulin, albumen and various monosaccharides and disaccharides are not excreted; from this it may be judged that filtration does not occur. Recent studies[77,118A] indicate that glucose is excreted by the aglomerular kidney, refuting earlier studies.

The mechanism utilized by aglomerular kidneys to form primary urine has not been studied directly. Presumably fluid is 'secreted' in a manner analogous to fluid secretion by Malpighian tubules (Chapters 7 and 8). The final urine of aglomerular fishes is qualitatively very similar to that of glomerular marine fishes. It is low in total concentration and in univalent ions. However, it is very meagre in volume.

In this review there has not been space enough to cover adequately all aspects of vertebrate renal physiology. Topics selected emphasize mechanisms which have some relevance to invertebrate renal physiology. Thus acid : base balance has been given little space and the juxtaglomerular apparatus has not been discussed at all. This is not to say that these subjects are unimportant to invertebrate renal physiology. However, it is difficult to assess the importance of subjects which have received virtually no attention from invertebrate renal physiologists. The renin : angiotensin system with which the juxtaglomerular apparatus of mammals and some lower vertebrates[32A] may be concerned intimately bears no relevance to invertebrates so far as it is known, but it would be surprising if an analogous system does not exist.

Part 3: Renal Function in Arthropods

Chapter 7

In arthropods two major types of renal organs are found: segmental organs which are derived from coelomoducts, and tubular organs which are derived as outpocketings of the gut.

Coelomoduct-derived renal organs

Coelomoduct renal organs are found in all arthropod groups, but they have been lost secondarily in the higher insects. They are called by various names, such as antennal glands, maxillary glands, labial glands, coxal glands and nephridia. The latter designation is inappropriate for reasons which will be discussed below. Coelomoduct renal organs consist of an end or coelomic sac (thought to represent a remnant of the coelom) and a tubule which leads to the outside of the body. In the renal organs of lower crustaceans and non-crustaceans, the tubule is usually simple. In higher crustaceans, the tubule is highly infolded; the folds anastomose so that the original tubule shape is lost.

Gut-derived renal organs

These organs arise as outpockets from the gut. Included here are Malpighian tubules and probably other 'tubules' which are called variously, 'digestive glands', 'digestive tubules' and 'gut appendages'. Only Malpighian tubules have been studied in any definitive way, so attention will be confined to those structures.

The Malpighian tubule–hindgut complex: an introduction

Malpighian tubules arise as outgrowths from the gut and form a functional unit with the posterior end of the gut. The number, location and gross morphology of the tubules vary widely in the arthropod groups. In myriapods and arachnids there appear to be only two;[140,205] in insects there are two to several hundred.[204] The end of the tubule distal to the gut lies free in the haemocoel, but in lepidopteran larvae and some beetles a so-called 'cryptonephridial' condition exists. The distal ends of the tubules are applied closely to the rectum and hindgut.

Malpighian tubules consist of flat or columnar cells which possess a brush border. It has been stated that the tubule cells of diplopods lack a brush border.[140] However, recent electron micrographs reveal that the Malpighian tubule cells of the millipede, *Glomeris marginata* possess uniform and scattered microvilli.[88A] The proximal ends of the Malpighian tubules may be expanded into ampullae in which the cells are columnar. In the insects, the Malpighian tubule cells are flat and quite large. The epithelium may be uniform throughout the tubule,[140] or it may be differentiated into two or more regions or cell types.[232]

The cells of the Malpighian tubules may be enclosed in a connective tissue sheath. Commonly there are spiral muscle strands within the sheath which impart a twisting, peristaltic movement to the tubules.

The foregoing generalized description of the anatomy of Malpighian tubules does not do justice to the wealth of information accumulated on the subject. Reviews by Palm[139,140] and Wigglesworth[232] should be consulted for more detailed information and references to other work.

The earliest and probably the best known of the electron microscopical studies of insect Malpighian tubules is that of Beams, Tahmisian and Devine[4] on the tubules of a grasshopper, *Melanoplus*; subsequent work has concentrated on details of ultrastructure or attempts to match ultrastructure with known function. Improvements in fixation and sectioning techniques as well as technical improvements in the electron microscope itself have served to increase resolution. Fig. 19 is a drawing of a survey (low power) electron micrograph of a tubule (primary) cell from the Malpighian tubules of the blowfly, *Calliphora erythrocephala* Meig. The basal area of the cell consists of a basement membrane and a cytoplasmic membrane. The latter infolds extensively into the interior of the cell. Between the infoldings are cytoplasmic compartments which contain mitochondria, dense bodies and other cellular inclusions. Scattered throughout the rest of the cytoplasm are more mitochondria, vacuoles and dense bodies. The apical region of the cell is bordered by the apical membrane which is thrown into a series of finger-like projections, the microvilli. In the diminished resolution of the light microscope, the microvillous border looks like a brush border. Protruding into most of the microvilli are elongate and sometimes branching mitochondria. This relationship of mitochondria and microvilli appears to be unique to the insects. It has been suggested that the positions of the mitochondria indicate that they flow into the microvilli and their bulbous ends are pinched off to lie free in the lumen.[4]

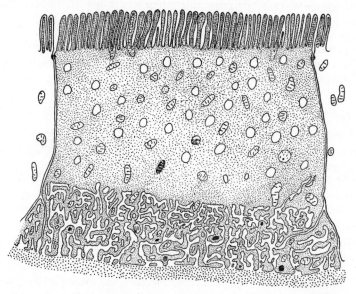

FIG. 19. Primary cell from Malpighian tubule of the blowfly, *Calliphora*. The microvilli contain mitochondria, some of which are branched. At the base of the cell are extensive channels. The cytoplasm is filled with mitochondria, 'vacuoles' and dense bodies of various kinds. Drawn from electron micrographs in Berridge and Oschman.[21]

Electron microscope studies have been made on the Malpighian tubules of a number of insects. However, the general arrangement seen in Fig. 21 is fairly characteristic of Malpighian tubules other than *Calliphora*. Therefore, unless ultrastructure materially helps to clarify some functional detail further discussion will not be made. Berridge and Oschman[21] have briefly reviewed work current to the time of writing this.

Renal function in myriapods and primitive insects

Studies of the function of Malpighian tubules, coelomoduct-derived renal organs (labial glands, coxal glands) and other tissues in myriapods and primitive insects concern their ability to accumulate or excrete dyes or other visible substances. These studies have been of little direct value to an understanding of the function of renal organs. So little is known about the physico-chemical characteristics of vital dyes that the fact that a tissue accumulates or releases them tells us little more than that. The value of such studies is that they identify organs and tissues which might prove interesting for further functional study. Further, many such studies provide valuable data on the microscopic structure of likely renal organs. The reader is referred to the studies of Feustel[48] on Collembola, and Palm[139,140] on insects and myriapods. The extensive studies of Lison[101] should be consulted for a resumé of studies of dye excretion and accumulation.

Renal function in the higher insects

Modern studies of insect renal physiology may be said to have begun with Wigglesworth's investigation of the blood-sucking bug, *Rhodnius prolixus* Stål. *Rhodnius* is an ideal insect for renal studies. After gorging itself with blood it undergoes a short-term diuresis during which it eliminates (through the rectum) most of the water gained during feeding. The copious fluid issuing from the rectum is almost entirely derived from the Malpighian tubules. After diuresis (three to four hours) the fluid flow diminishes; after about the first day, no fluid is voided from the rectum.

Wigglesworth[230] analyzed fluid voided during the diuretic phase, as well as the rectal contents over the ensuing days when no fluid was voided. From these analyses and other observations he formed two main conclusions regarding excretion in *Rhodnius*. 1. During the first day after feeding, the bug eliminates substances which are derived from the blood meal and excreted unaltered. These are water, sodium, potassium, calcium, magnesium (*sic*), chloride, carbonate, phosphate and probably urea. 2. Subsequent to the first day, uric acid, sulphate and creatine are eliminated, presumably as end-products of the bug's metabolism; the Malpighian tubules continue to secrete fluid into the rectum, but most of the water is reabsorbed there.

The Malpighian tubules of *Rhodnius* consist of a clear upper segment and an opaque lower segment. The opacity of the lower (proximal) segment is due to the presence of uric acid crystals in the lumen. Wigglesworth concluded that the uric acid crystals were in the form of acid potassium urate.

From his observations on *Rhodnius*, Wigglesworth concluded that there is a constant circulation of water and base between the haemolymph and Malpighian tubules. Water and acid potassium urate are secreted into the upper segment. The acid potassium urate is converted to uric acid in the lower segment. The base and water are then reabsorbed and the uric acid, being insoluble, precipitates out of solution.

Wigglesworth[231] went on to investigate the relationships of Malpighian tubules and hindguts in insects representing several insect orders. He concluded that the Malpighian tubule and hindgut represent a complex through which water circulates. That is, water which enters the Malpighian tubules may be reabsorbed in the tubules, or rectum or both (e.g. *Rhodnius*). Not all insects investigated by Wigglesworth had uric acid crystals in the Malpighian tubules. Further, in some (e.g. Diptera) uric acid crystals were found to occupy the whole of the lumen of the tubules. In these insects, he suggested, the mechanism for the precipitation of uric acid may be different than in *Rhodnius*.

Studies made subsequent to those of Wigglesworth indicate that end-products of nitrogen metabolism other than uric acid are eliminated, sometimes in significant quantities. These include urea, allantoin and amino acids.

In most insects, the renal system (Malpighian tubules, hindgut/rectum) is connected to the alimentary tract. It is therefore difficult to discern the roles of the individual parts of the system merely by collecting material from the rectum of intact animals. The fluid issuing from the rectum of *Rhodnius* during the diuretic phase is probably entirely the product of the Malpighian tubules. However, *Rhodnius* is a special case. Another special case is the cotton stainer, *Dysdercus fasciatus* Signoret, in which the midgut and rectum are not connected during the larval stages; material collected from the rectal aperture is all derived from the Malpighian tubules.[12] The obvious way to get round the difficulty of separating tubule and rectal function is to make direct studies of the tissues in isolation from each other. That is, they may be separated physically or functionally from the rest of the insect's body. This has had great success in a number of cases which will now be examined.

Direct studies of Malpighian tubules: 'early' studies

It was mentioned in Chapter 2 that perhaps the greatest difficulty in making direct studies of renal function is that of analyzing the small amounts of fluid obtainable by micropuncture. Therefore, renal physiology owes a debt to Professor J. A. Ramsay and his colleagues, R. H. J. Brown, S. W. H. W. Falloon and P. C. Croghan. They are responsible for the design and development of ingenious instrumental methods for the analysis of osmotic pressure, sodium and potassium, and chloride in nannolitre amounts of biological fluids.

Study of the Malpighian tubules of Rhodnius

Two major questions which Wigglesworth was unable to answer were investigated by Ramsay in his study of excretion in Rhodnius[161] 1. Do sodium and potassium concentrations in the Malpighian tubule fluid and haemolymph of *Rhodnius* vary independently? 2. Do the upper and lower segments of the tubules carry out distinctive roles in the excretion of sodium and potassium?

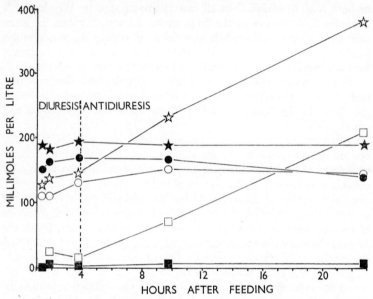

FIG. 20.   Urine (rectal fluid) and haemolymph osmotic pressures, and concentrations of sodium and potassium, in *Rhodnius*, for a period of about one day after feeding. Open stars = urine osmotic pressure; closed stars = haemolymph osmotic pressure; open circles = urine sodium concentration; closed circles = haemolymph sodium concentration; open squares = urine potassium concentration; closed squares = haemolymph potassium concentration. From Ramsay.[161]

Ramsay followed changes in osmotic pressure and concentrations of sodium and potassium in the haemolymph and rectal fluid of insects fed normally on rabbit's blood. Figure 20 illustrates the changes in osmotic pressure and concentrations of sodium and potassium in the urine and haemolymph of a specimen of *Rhodnius* during 24 hours following a normal meal. The excretory system is able to maintain the haemolymph relatively constant with respect to the measured parameters. This answered Ramsay's first question; the sodium and potassium concentrations in the urine and haemolymph do vary independently of each other. These studies showed also that considerable water and sodium are reabsorbed from the urine, whilst relatively less potassium is reabsorbed (Fig. 20).

In further experiments, the haemolymph potassium concentration was artificially elevated by allowing the insects to feed on ox blood to which potassium chloride was added. For the first day after feeding the insects maintained the blood potassium concentrations at relatively low levels. It appeared that this success was due to the activities of the Malpighian tubules. However, after the first day, for some reason, regulation of the haemolymph potassium concentration failed and the animals died slowly.

Subsequent studies have shown that Malpighian tubules isolated from *Rhodnius* are able to function when bathed in a medium whose potassium concentration is considerably higher than that shown in Fig. 20. This illustrates what is probably the major advantage of studying tissues in isolation. The morbidity of the specimens of *Rhodnius* in Ramsay's experiments was undoubtedly due to factors not related to the Malpighian tubules, but study of the function of those structures was frustrated by the lesser tolerance of other tissues for high potassium concentration in the haemolymph.

Ramsay sampled the upper and lower segments of the Malpighian tubules of *Rhodnius*. He compared the tubular fluid to the haemolymph with respect to the sodium and potassium concentrations and osmotic pressures. The average values obtained are shown in Table 12. These results indicated that the upper portion of the Malpighian tubule of

TABLE 12

Concentrations of sodium and potassium and the osmotic pressure of the haemolymph and Malpighian tubule fluid of Rhodnius *fed on a normal diet and on a high-potassium diet. The normal diet was rabbit's blood. The high-potassium diet was ox blood augmented with potassium chloride. Data from Ramsay.*[161]

	Haemolymph			Upper tubule			Lower tubule		
	Na	K	OP	Na	K	OP	Na	K	OP
Normal diet	169	7	200	128	86	233	167	43	212
High K diet	150	18	181	79	144	224	92	106	182

Rhodnius elaborates a fluid which is higher in osmotic pressure and potassium concentration but contains less sodium than does the haemolymph. In the lower tubule the fluid becomes more like the haemolymph, except that the potassium concentration remains high. The results of these experiments answered Ramsay's second question: the upper and

D

lower portions of the Malpighian tubule of *Rhodnius* do carry on distinctive functions.

Wigglesworth concluded that fluid is reabsorbed in the lower portion of the tubule. The results of Ramsay's study neither supported nor refuted this, but they did indicate that if fluid is reabsorbed in the lower tubule it may be due to some active mechanism. The fluid entering the lower tubule from the upper tubule (Table 12) has a higher osmotic pressure than the haemolymph. Fluid reabsorption which occurs in the lower tubule must proceed against an osmotic gradient, which would imply that it is active.

Active potassium transport by the insect Malpighian tubule

In order to ascertain the ubiquity of potassium secretion by Malpighian tubules, Ramsay[162] studied sodium and potassium concentrations in the haemolymph and tubule fluid in several insects. These included specimens of eight species representing five orders. In all, the potassium concentration of the Malpighian tubule fluid exceeded the potassium concentration of the haemolymph (Table 13). Additionally, he measured transtubular electrical potentials. As discussed in Chapter 2, it is not sufficient to have knowledge of the ion concentration gradients across epithelia; some knowledge of the electrical relationships must be gained before it can be judged whether or not active transport of a particular ion occurs.

The high potassium concentrations in the tubule fluid of the insects could be due to the retention of that ion in the lumen by a large negative potential. Using the Nernst equation (Chapter 2, p. 13) Ramsay

TABLE 13

Electrical potential differences measured (pd_meas) across the Malpighian tubules of various insects (1), potential differences calculated by the Nernst equation (pd_eq) from transtubular sodium and potassium concentrations (2 and 3), and algebraic differences between the measured and calculated potential differences (4 and 5). All values are in millivolts and the sign refers to the tubule lumen. From Ramsay.[162]

	1	2 Na	3 K	4 Na	5 K
Insect	pd_{meas}	pd_{eq}	pd_{eq}	$pd_{eq} - pd_{meas}$	$pd_{eq} - pd_{meas}$
Locusta	−16	+5	−46	+21	−30
Dixippus*	+21	+23	−55	+2	−76
Pieris	+28	+9	−45	−19	−73
Tenebrio	+45	+36	−47	−9	−92
Dytiscus	+22	+29	−86	+7	−108
A tabanid	—	+45	−87	—	—
Rhodnius	−35	+7	−72	+42	−37
Aedes	+21	+32	−85	+11	−106

* Now designated as *Carausius*.

calculated the electrical potential differences at equilibrium (pd_{eq}) which could account for the observed differences in the concentrations of sodium and potassium between the haemolymph and tubule fluid. The measured potential differences (pd_{meas}) were then subtracted (algebraically) from the calculated values. If the result of this calculation was negative, then active transport was assumed.

In no case (Table 13) was the potassium concentration difference between the tubule fluid and haemolymph explicable in terms of the measured electrical potential difference. Therefore, the distribution of potassium was considered to be due to an active process. From the foregoing it was concluded that it is very likely that active secretion of potassium into the Malpighian tubule is a general phenomenon in insects. Secretion of sodium may also occur, but the data were too variable to place great reliance upon them.

Studies on the isolated Malpighian tubules of the stick insect

A major drawback to the study of renal function in arthropods is their possession of an 'open' circulatory system. This makes it technically difficult to expose the interior of the animals without major physiological changes occurring, the haemolymph may clot or the haemocoelar hydrostatic pressure may become depressed. To obviate these difficulties, Wigglesworth sealed the opening he made in *Rhodnius* with a coverslip. Ramsay worked rapidly, but in both cases the experiments were hampered.

Ramsay developed a technique in which Malpighian tubules could be isolated in a drop of haemolymph or Ringer under liquid paraffin (mineral oil), an inert material immiscible with water. This technique represented a major breakthrough in the study of insect excretion, and it is still the basis of most recent studies of Malpighian tubule function. In a series of studies, Ramsay[163-167] established the 'secretion-diffusion' theory of urine formation in insects, which stands today. This work was done using females of the stick insect, *Carausius morosus*, which are reared easily in the laboratory and are very large (75 to 100 millimetres in length).

In *Carausius* potassium is transported actively into the Malpighian tubule. The fluid produced at the proximal (to the gut) end of the isolated tubules normally is slightly hypoosmotic to the haemolymph, suggesting that water may be transported actively into the tubule. However, this view was proved to be untenable in subsequent studies. It could be established that the rate of urine formation was directly correlated with the haemolymph potassium concentration (Fig. 21). When the serum (haemolymph from which protein was removed by

heat coagulation) potassium concentration was elevated there was an
increase in fluid production. It was demonstrated that sodium could
enter the tubules against an electrochemical gradient, although the
haemolymph normally has a higher sodium concentration than does
the tubule fluid. When the haemolymph (serum) potassium concentration was reduced to very low levels, the concentration of sodium in
the tubule fluid exceeded that in the serum. There appeared to
be no competition between sodium and potassium for transport into
the tubule lumen.

A feature of all Malpighian tubules studied by Ramsay was the
elevated tubule fluid potassium concentration. That this situation was
brought about by active cellular metabolism in all cases was undoubted.

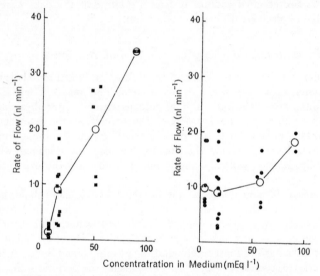

FIG. 21.   Rate of fluid production by isolated Malpighian
tubules of *Carausius* when potassium (squares) and sodium
(circles) are the major cations in the bathing medium. From
Ramsay.[165]

However, the significance of this relationship to a general theory of
fluid production by Malpighian tubules was not clear. The results of
the study of the Malpighian tubules of *Rhodnius* would seem to indicate
that active potassium secretion into the tubule elevates the osmotic
pressure of the tubular fluid. Water (and diffusible solutes) would then
tend to move into the tubules passively. That this situation might not
pertain to *Carausius* was obvious. The osmotic pressure of the tubule
fluid is usually slightly less than the osmotic pressure of the haemolymph.

The alternative to a passive flow of fluid generated by an osmotic gradient was the hypothesis that each individual metabolite is secreted by an active mechanism. If metabolites move from the medium into the tubule fluid directly due to the active metabolism of the cells, then some point must be reached where the transfer mechanism ('carrier') is saturated. At this point the concentration of the metabolities in the tubule fluid will diminish relative to the concentration of the metabolites in the medium.

Ramsay tested this hypothesis for the following metabolites: calcium, magnesium, chloride, phosphate, hydrogen ion, glycine, arginine, alanine, lysine, proline, valine, urea, glucose, fructose, sucrose and inulin. With the exception of phosphate and urea, all substances tested were substantially less concentrated in the tubule fluid than in the medium. Phosphate was more concentrated in the tubule fluid than in the medium. Urea was equally concentrated in tubule fluid and medium. However, in no case could it be established that movement of substances into the tubule lumen from the medium was limited or saturated. In some cases, such as sugars, there was evidence that the substances were partially metabolized passing from the medium to the tubule lumen.

A very conclusive argument for diffusion of organic compounds from serum to tubule lumen arose from work with mixtures of amino acids and a mixture of an amino acid, glucose and urea. The tubule fluid : medium ratios (TF/M) of amino acids, urea and glucose when present in the medium in mixtures were similar to the TF/M when the organic compounds were present individually in the medium. Thus there was no apparent competition between related or unrelated compounds for transport into the tubule lumen.

A final experiment demonstrated that a diffusive process most probably underlies passage of organic compounds into the Malpighian tubule lumen. Tubules were set up as depicted in Fig. 22. The main body of each tubule was put into a large droplet of medium (3) containing radioactive urea or sucrose. A second smaller droplet of medium (1) was placed some distance from the first drop. The second droplet did not contain the organic compound under test. After four hours, the fluid produced (2) and the second droplet (1) were collected and their radio-activity measured. The results (tabular insert to Fig. 22), showed that most of the urea and sucrose in the tubular fluid passed out of the lumen into the second droplet (1). Both substances, sucrose and urea, can pass through the tubule wall in both directions; this evidence strongly supports the view that diffusion underlies passage of organic molecules across the Malpighian tubule epithelium. Of course, these experiments did not ascertain that the rate of diffusion was the same in both directions.

On the basis of his studies, Ramsay postulated a theory of urine formation in the insect Malpighian tubule which has come to be known as the 'secretion-diffusion' theory. Briefly, this hypothesis envisages that potassium is transported actively (secreted) into the tubule lumen. This establishes a flow of fluid which carries all diffusible substances across the tubule epithelium. The permeability of the tubule epithelium

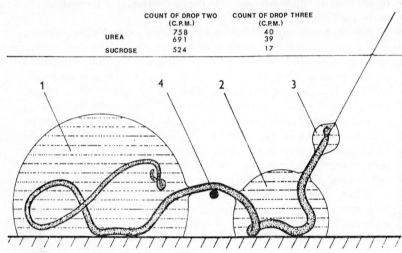

	COUNT OF DROP TWO (C.P.M.)	COUNT OF DROP THREE (C.P.M.)
UREA	758 691	40 39
SUCROSE	524	17

FIG. 22. Measurement of two-way permeability to urea and sucrose of the isolated Malpighian tubule of *Carausius*. Radioactive sucrose or urea is placed in the medium (1) and its concentration in a second drop of medium (2) and in the fluid produced by the tubule (3) is measured after a suitable interval. The tubule is supported in the liquid paraffin by a rod (4). *Inset table*: concentration of urea and sucrose (in counts per minute) in drops 2 and 3 after an experiment was terminated. From Ramsay.[167]

determines the actual amount of diffusible substances which enter the urine. Thus the most permeable substance tested was urea. Here the concentration of the tubule fluid was always about equal to the concentration in the medium. The least permeable substance tested was inulin.* Its concentration in the tubular fluid was only about 1/20th the concentration in the medium.[169]

* Recent studies suggest that all Malpighian tubules may not be so impermeable to inulin as those of *Carausius*. The concentration of inulin in fluid produced by isolated tubules of *Calliphora* averages 46% of the medium concentration (i.e., $TF/M = 0.46$)[146A]. Furthermore, the inulin tubule fluid: medium concentration ratio in fluid produced by Malpighian tubules isolated from the millipede, *Glomeris*, may exceed one although the average TF/M equals 0.68.[88A]

Chapter 8

Recent studies of isolated Malpighian tubules

A most significant recent finding in the study of insect Malpighian tubules is the ability of some to survive and function in an apparently healthy state in artificial media. Malpighian tubules of four species of insects have been studied in this way. These are: the entire tubules of the blowfly, *Calliphora* [14,16,17] and the stick insect, *Carausius*,[149] the non-cryptonephridial portions of the tubules of the larvae of the water skimmer, *Calpodes ethlius* Stoll[83] and the upper portion of the tubules of *Rhodnius*.[114] The tubules of *Carausius* and *Rhodnius* produce fluid maximally in the presence of a 'diuretic' factor derived from parts of the nervous system.

The ability of Malpighian tubules to function in artificial media offers enormous experimental advantages; the bathing medium may be defined with relative precision; metabolites can be added or deleted and their concentrations in the medium can be varied over a large range. Although almost all tubules will function in a medium composed only of Ringer plus glucose, for long-term health and function complex organic compounds must be included.

In recent studies the role that the tubules play in fluid and ion transport has taken precedence over their role in the economy of the insect. However, it is reasonable to expect that as knowledge accumulates it will be possible to put the tubules back into the insect, so to speak.

Fluid and solute transport by Malpighian tubules

The effect of osmotic pressure on fluid transport. Probably the only feature shared by all isolated Malpighian tubules is the utter dependence of fluid production on the osmotic pressure of the suspending medium. Fig. 23 illustrates the inverse relationship between the osmotic pressure of the medium and the rate of fluid production in *Rhodnius*.[114] However, with minor modifications the figure could serve also to illustrate the phenomenon in *Carausius*,[165] *Dysdercus*,[13] *Calliphora*[16] and *Calpodes*.[83] The underlying cause of this relationship is not clear.

The effect of ions on fluid and ion transport. Transport of sodium across the tubule epithelium seems to be mirrored by the transport of potassium (Fig. 24). When fluid produced by the tubules has a high potassium concentration, the sodium concentration is low, and vice versa. This may be due to two factors, the availability of ions for transport and the selectivity of the transport mechanism for specific ions.

When sodium in the medium is in low concentration, potassium is preferentially transported; when the potassium concentration in the

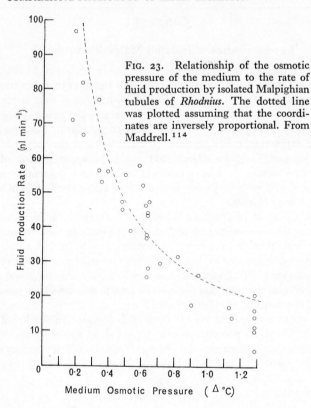

FIG. 23. Relationship of the osmotic pressure of the medium to the rate of fluid production by isolated Malpighian tubules of *Rhodnius*. The dotted line was plotted assuming that the coordinates are inversely proportional. From Maddrell.[114]

medium is low, sodium is preferentially transported (Fig. 24). It seems as if some ion must be transported and if the preferred ion species is not available, substitutions can be made, within limits. Whilst either sodium or potassium can be transported by isolated tubules, very different fluid production rates result when only one or the other ion is present in the medium. As shown in Table 14, only a meagre flow of fluid occurs when all of the potassium in the medium bathing tubules of *Calliphora* is replaced by sodium. Under the same circumstances the isolated tubules of *Rhodnius* produce fluid at maximum rates. When all the sodium in the bathing medium is replaced by potassium, the isolated tubules of *Calliphora* produce fluid at a maximum rate. Under the same conditions the tubules of *Rhodnius* produce fluid at a greatly reduced rate.

The isolated tubules of *Calliphora* are highly selective for potassium. When they are producing fluid slowly in a medium in which all the potassium has been replaced by sodium, the rates of fluid production and potassium transport (Fig. 24) both jump abruptly when only 8 mM l⁻¹ potassium is added. Thereafter, the rates of fluid production and potassium transport are linearly related to the concentration of potassium in the medium. Furthermore, the rate of sodium transport is low relative to potassium transport rate, resulting in a decreasing concentration of sodium in the tubule fluid. The isolated tubules of

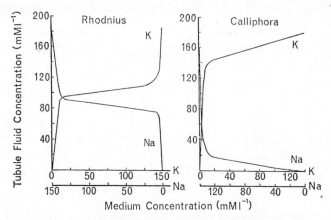

FIG. 24. Effects of replacement of sodium in the medium by potassium, and vice versa, on the concentration of sodium and potassium in fluid produced by isolated Malpighian tubules of *Rhodnius* and *Calliphora*. From Maddrell.[114]

TABLE 14

Fluid production rates of Malpighian tubules isolated in media in which the major cations are those listed.

Cation	Calliphora* Flow Rate (nl min⁻¹)	Rhodnius** Flow Rate (Percent of Control Ringer)
Control Ringer***	—	100
Potassium	13·8	40
Sodium	0·4	90—100
Rubidium	10·9	—
Ammonium	0	35—40
Caesium	2·5	—
Lithium	0	—
Tetraethyl Ammonium (TEA)	—	0·1
Choline	0	0·1

    * Data from Berridge.[16]

  ** Data from Maddrell.[114]

*** *Rhodnius* Ringer containing glucose and diuretic hormone.

Rhodnius are not so selective for either sodium or potassium. The tubule fluid concentrations of sodium and potassium are similar except when one ion is much more concentrated than the other ion in the medium; of course sodium transport is paralleled by a fluid transport rate which is more rapid than is the case when potassium is being transported (Fig. 24).

Selectivity for ions by isolated Malpighian tubules is not limited to sodium and potassium. Significant fluid production rates occur when

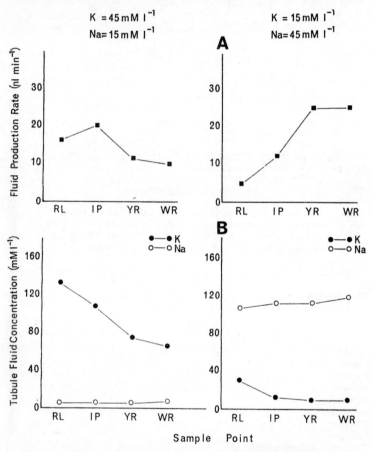

FIG. 25.   Effect of high potassium, low sodium and high sodium, low potassium media on the fluid production rate (**A**) and concentrations of sodium and potassium (**B**) in fluid produced by different segments of the isolated Malpighian tubules of *Calpodes*. RL = rectal lead; IP = iliac plexus; YR = yellow region; WR = white region. From Irvine.[83]

sodium and potassium in the medium bathing the tubules of *Calliphora* are replaced by rubidium and caesium (Table 14). Isolated tubules of *Rhodnius* produce fluid in a medium in which sodium and potassium have been replaced by ammonium ion.

In common with other fluid-transporting tissues, isolated Malpighian tubules will not produce fluid in the presence of large concentrations of poorly-penetrating ions, such as choline (Table 14). However, when only small amounts of transportable ions (sodium or potassium) are added to the choline medium, fluid production begins and thereafter the rate varies linearly with the concentration of transportable ions in the medium.[15,16,114]

An interesting variation on the pattern seen previously is presented by the studies of Irvine,[83] on segments of the Malpighian tubules of larval *Calpodes*. The tubules could be divided into four morphologically-distinct parts. From distal to proximal (to the gut) these are the rectal lead (*RL*), iliac plexus (*IP*), yellow region (*YR*) and white region (*WR*). Alteration of the ratios of sodium and potassium in the bathing medium altered the site of fluid production in the isolated tubules (Fig. 25a); simultaneously, the concentrations of sodium and potassium in the fluid produced was altered (Fig. 25b). It appears that the upper (distal) parts (*RL* + *IP*) of the tubules preferentially transport sodium, whilst the lower (proximal) parts (*YR* + *WR*) preferentially transport potassium.

Either phosphate or chloride (but not both) may accumulate in the fluid produced by isolated Malpighian tubules. Chloride is highly concentrated (relative to the medium) in fluid produced by isolated tubules of *Rhodnius*.[114] Phosphate is highly concentrated (relative to the medium) in fluid produced by isolated tubules of *Carausius* and *Calliphora*.[17,166] Accumulation of phosphate and chloride may be due to active mechanisms, but the nature of these mechanisms has not been discovered. Probably all other anions enter the tubule fluid passively; their concentration depends upon their hydrated radius. Fig. 26 compares the hydrated radii of a large number of anions with the fluid production rates that they will sustain. With the exception of phosphate, which may be transported actively, the larger the anion, the less rapid the fluid production rate it will sustain.

Metabolic events underlying fluid production by isolated Malpighian tubules

Little is known about the metabolic events which directly or indirectly underlie fluid production by Malpighian tubules. The isolated-tubule preparation has permitted a direct approach to this problem through the use of metabolites and inhibitors.

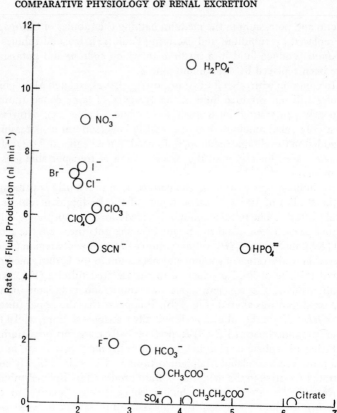

FIG. 26. Fluid production rates of isolated Malpighian tubules of *Calliphora* in media in which the dominant anions are those illustrated. The fluid production rates are compared with the hydrated radii of the dominant anions. From Berridge.[17]

Metabolites. High rates of fluid production were sustained by isolated Malpighian tubules of *Calliphora* when their medium contained metabolites drawn from all of the following catagories: Monosaccharides, oligosaccharides, phosphorylated compounds, pyruvate, Krebs cycle acids and amino acids. Some compounds in each catagory were either incapable of supporting fluid production or they caused fluid to be produced slowly. There was no obvious physical difference (e.g. molecular weight) between many of the compounds; this observation possibly ruled out differential rates of diffusion across the tubule wall as a factor.

For example, maltose would support a high rate of fluid production whilst lactose, a molecule of the same size, would not. If Ramsay's suggestion[167] that organic molecules enter the tubule lumen by diffusion is correct, the two sugars should support equal rates of fluid production. It was suggested by Berridge that the compounds which would support high rates of fluid production entered into the metabolism of the cells.

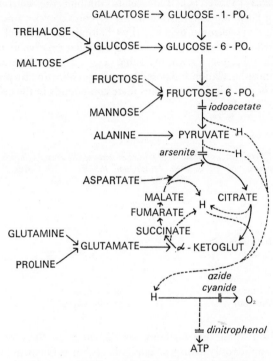

FIG. 27. Possible metabolic pathways in cells of the Malpighian tubules of *Calliphora*. Also shown are inhibitors, and their postulated places of action. From Berridge.[14]

If this assumption is correct, then it is possible to gain insight into the metabolic events which underlie Malpighian tubule function.

Malpighian tubule cells possibly derive energy for fluid production from glycolytic-Krebs cycle pathways; compounds which feed directly into those cycles appeared to be most effective in promoting fluid production (see Fig. 27). However, it may be recalled that monosaccharide uptake by the proximal tubules of the vertebrate nephron (Chapter 5) appears to depend upon the structural configuration of the transported molecule. It is possible that the same is true in Malpighian tubules. Therefore, molecules of the same size and molecular weight may be transported differentially because of molecular configurational differences.

Inhibitors. The chemical inhibitors, iodoacetate, cyanide and azide block fluid production by the isolated tubules of both *Calliphora* and *Rhodnius* (Table 15). Iodoacetate inhibits the conversion of fructose-6-phosphate to pyruvate in the glycolytic cycle; cyanide and azide inhibit cytochrome oxidase, thus halting the terminal reaction in the electron-transfer chain and halting aerobic oxidative metabolism. The fourth inhibitor shown in Table 15, 2,4-dinitrophenol, stops oxidative phosphorylation and possibly expresses its action by preventing the supply of new high-energy phosphate compounds in the cells of the Malpighian tubules.

TABLE 15

Effectiveness of various inhibitors in slowing the rate of fluid production by isolated Malpighian tubules of Rhodnius. From Maddrell.[114]

Inhibitor	Concentration $(M \, l^{-1})$ reducing fluid flow rate by 50 per cent.
Cyanide	3×10^{-4}
Iodoacetate	3×10^{-3}
Azide	10^{-3}
2,4-dinitrophenol	10^{-5}
Copper ions	$3 \cdot 5 \times 10^{-5}$
Acetazolamide	no effect at 10^{-2}
Ouabain	no effect at 10^{-3}

The observation that ouabain has no effect on fluid production (Table 15) applies only to insect Malpighian tubules. Ouabain halts fluid production by Malpighian tubules isolated from the pill millipede *Glomeris*. The reason for this difference is not clear. Malpighian tubules of *Glomeris* produce fluid which is almost isosmotic with the bathing medium and neither sodium nor potassium are concentrated.[88A] It is argued that ouabain exerts its effect by inhibiting sodium- and potassium-activated adenosine triphosphatase (ATPase), thus halting sodium and potassium transport. However, such is not the case in insects, and it is likely that an alternative explanation for the effect of ouabain or function of ATPase must be found.

Copper ions inhibit the movement of chloride into Malpighian tubules (Table 15, Fig. 28). It is rather puzzling that copper should inhibit the tubules of both *Rhodnius* and *Calliphora*. In the former,

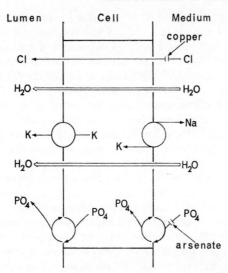

FIG. 28.   Model of fluid production proposed for the Malpighian tubules of *Calliphora*. Potassium is transported
actively into the cell from the medium at the basal membrane in exchange for sodium, which diffuses into the cell.
At the apical border potassium is pumped into the lumen,
possibly electrogenically (i.e. without a charge-balancing
counter ion). Phosphate moves across both the basal and
apical membranes of the cell by some kind of carrier. Water
moves passively across the cell down an osmotic gradient
established by active potassium transport. Anions (chloride
illustrated) move passively across the cell through pores
which may be blocked by copper ions. Modified from
Berridge.[15]

chloride is thought to be transported actively; in the latter, it appears
to move passively. It is thought that copper exerts its well-known
effect by blocking 'pores' through which anions move passively.

Concentration of phosphate by isolated tubules of *Calliphora* can
be blocked by arsenate, a molecule whose structure is similar to that of
phosphate. It is thought that arsenate competitively inhibits phosphate
transport.

Summary and discussion of fluid production by isolated Malpighian tubules

In the current view water and most solutes move passively across
fluid-transporting epithelia driven by the active transport of a few
solutes (Chapter 12). The solutes of greatest importance to this process

are sodium and potassium. It is clear that no single scheme will suffice to explain fluid production by all isolated Malpighian tubules. However, this probably only reflects that lack of breadth, if not depth, of current knowledge. Berridge (Fig. 28) has put forward a scheme which may suffice for the tubules of *Calliphora*, and probably *Carausius* as well: a sodium : potassium exchange pump may be present on the basal membrane of the Malpighian tubule cell, which pumps potassium into the cell in exchange for sodium which diffuses into the cell. On the apical membrane of the cell is a pump which transports potassium from the cell into the lumen, possibly setting up an electrical potential across the tubule epithelium. The apical pump could be 'electrogenic'. That is, it may separate charge by pumping only potassium without a counter ion.

The presence of a sodium : potassium exchange pump on the basal membrane of the cell would explain why fluid production slows in media containing little potassium. The apical potassium pump must then depend upon the (relatively slow) diffusion of potassium into the cell. Phosphate ions are transported across the cell by carriers located on both the apical and basal membranes. All other anions diffuse across the cell in relation to their size, suggesting that the cells membranes have pores.

Sodium and potassium transport by isolated tubules of *Rhodnius* may be due to quite a different process involving movement of sodium and potassium across the tubule by two steps in series. The first step involves a 'cooperative' pump which allows sodium and potassium to enter the cell more quickly when both are present in the medium. This pump could be coupled to a second pump which preferentially transports sodium, but will transport potassium when sodium is in low concentration.

The basic thesis of the secretion-diffusion theory proposed by Ramsay, suitably modified to take account of recent studies, still stands. However, as yet there is still little conclusive evidence for the mechanism underlying movement of potassium (or sodium) into the tubule lumen. Berridge and Oschman[21] have proposed a scheme of fluid transport by Malpighian tubules based on the filtration of small particles by the basement membrane of the tubule cells, which will be considered in Chapter 12.

Hormonal control of tubule function

Several studies have implicated 'hormones' from various parts of the insect nervous system in the control of excretion. For example, experiments of Wall[222] and Wall and Ralph[224] suggest that an antidiuretic principle is produced in the supraoesophageal ganglion (brain) and stored in the *corpora allata* of the cockroach, *Periplaneta americana* L. Further, extracts of the nervous system of *Carausius*, purified by chromatography, affect the absorption rate of various dyes by the Malpighian tubules.[218] Extracts from many parts of the nervous system have a diuretic effect on isolated Malpighian tubules of *Dysdercus*.[13] Extracts of the corpora cardiaca increase fluid production by the isolated tubules of *Carausius*.[149]

Further remarks on hormonal effects on Malpighian tubule function will be confined to a review of studies by Maddrell,[108-112] which are easily the least equivocal. Maddrell's studies have revealed a detailed picture of the mode of release, action and fate of the diuretic hormone in *Rhodnius*. The reader is recommended to read Maddrell's papers, if only to discover for himself the sheer elegance of the experimental method when properly applied.

It will be recalled that *Rhodnius* gorges itself with blood and excretes most of the water in the meal within a few hours after feeding. The blood meal mechanically distorts the abdomen. Stretch receptors in the tergosternal muscles are triggered due to the upward displacement of the tergum (dorsal side of the abdomenal wall). Impulses from the tergosternal stretch receptors travel to the mesothoracic ganglionic mass, stimulating the release of the diuretic hormone. The hormone is produced in special neurosecretory cells in the mesothoracic ganglionic mass and travels to release (neurohaemal) sites via the abdomenal nerves. The hormone is released in quantities a little in excess of those required to promote maximum tubule activity. It is deactivated by the Malpighian tubules so that fluid production halts soon after release of the hormone is slowed. The neurohumour, 5-hydroxytryptamine mimics the action of the diuretic hormone in *Rhodnius*,[115] but not in *Carausius*.[113] Unlike the diuretic hormone, however, 5-HT is not deactivated by the Malpighian tubules.

The insect hindgut and rectum

The Malpighian tubules are only half of a renal system, the half which is responsible for removing materials from the haemolymph. The hindgut and/or rectum form the other half of the excretory system. They are responsible for the recovery of water and reabsorbable solutes which enter from the Malpighian tubules and alimentary canal. In the majority of terrestrial insects the rectal material is solid or semi-solid, depending upon the hydration state of the animal. A number of studies have indicated that the rectum is the main site of water reabsorption (see reference 18).

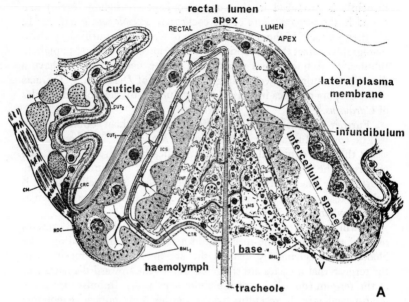

FIG. 29. *Above*: A. Fine structure of a rectal papilla of the blowfly, *Calliphora* schematic. *Opposite*: B. Fine structure of the rectal complex of the mealworm, *Tenebrio* schematic. C. Gross anatomy of the rectal complex of *Tenebrio*. A, from Gupta and Berridge,[71] B, C, from Ramsay.[168]

The structure of the rectum. In many insects the rectal surface is increased by specialized thickenings of the epithelial wall, which form pads or papillae. In many beetles (Coleoptera) and the larvae of Lepidoptera the distal ends of the Malpighian tubules are closely applied to the outside of the rectum, forming a 'rectal complex'.

The rectal lumen is bounded by a cuticle which is continuous with the exoskeleton. The rectal epithelium is composed of columnar cells; where the rectal epithelium is thrown into pads or papillae a very complex structural arrangement may be found. The ultrastructural details of the rectal papillae of the blowfly are illustrated in Fig. 29A. The papilla is divided into cortical and medullary regions. The cortex contains the epidermal cells and fine ramifications of the tracheoles. The border of the cortical cells, just under the cuticular intima, is thrown into microvillous-like apical leaflets. The lateral plasma membrane of the epidermal cells is elaborated into very extensive intercellular spaces. The cortical region is separated from the medullary region by the infundibular space. The intercellular and infundibular spaces are

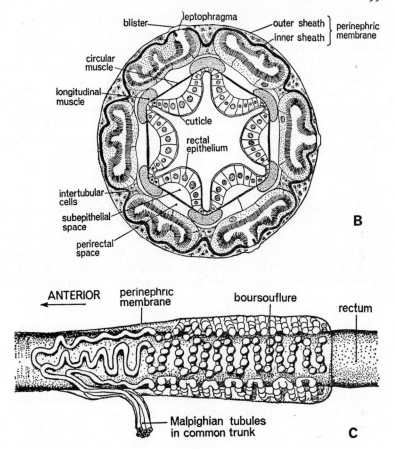

separated from the haemocoel by valve-like structures. Not shown in the figure are peculiar tightly-stacked membranes which appear to open to the intercellular spaces of the cortical cells.

Figure 29C illustrates the salient features of the rectal complex of the mealworm, *Tenebrio molitor* L. The distal ends of the six Malpighian tubules are closely applied to the rectum. The dorsal sides of the tubules form bubble-shaped structures or '*boursouflures*'. At the apex of each *boursouflure* is what appears to be an opening, the leptophragma. In reality it is only a thin area of the Malpighian tubule which is occupied by a special type of cell, the leptophragma cell (Fig. 29B). Completely surrounding the complex is the perinephric membrane. Where this membrane overlies the leptophragmata blisters are formed.

The rectal complex give rise to a number of spaces which are separated from the haemolymph by membranes or epithelia (Fig. 29B). From outside to inside these are the lumen of the Malpighian tubule, the perirectal space, the subepithelial space of the rectal epithelium and the rectal lumen.

The fine structure of the cells of the rectal epithelium are similar to those illustrated in Fig. 29A. Instead of membranous stacks at the lateral cell membranes there are numerous microtubules. The cells of the Malpighian tubule component of the rectal complex are similar to the cells of other Malpighian tubules (Fig. 19, p. 77). Most of the microvilli at the apical borders of the cells contain mitochondria. The basal region of the cells is occupied by membranous infoldings, but these lack mitochondria between them. The leptophragma cells bear widely-spaced microvilli. Part of each cell is produced into a plate-like structure which forms the leptophragma proper (Fig. 29B).

The structure of the rectal pads of the cockroach, *Periplaneta* has been studied by Wall and Oschman[223] (Fig. 33). The epithelium of the pads is columnar. The lateral cell membranes are greatly folded. Numerous mitochondria are seen in the cytoplasm between the folds. There are also intercellular channels between the lateral margins of the cells which are closed apically and basally by septate desmosomes. The intercellular channels occasionally widen to form dilations. Here and there the basal cell surface indents, forming a space into which a tracheal branch extends. Near the apical surface of the rectal cells large intercellular spaces communicate with both the intercellular channels and the basal indentations. The apical surface of the cells is highly folded and mitochondria are found between the folds. The apical side of the rectal epithelial cells is bounded by a cuticular intima, outside of which lies the rectal lumen. The basal surface of the rectal pad epithelium is bounded by a muscular sheath; between this and the basement membrane of the epithelium lies the subepithelial space or sinus. Communication between the subepithelial sinus and the haemolymph may occur through openings which are closed by one-way valves.

The function of the rectum. The work of Wigglesworth[230] demonstrated that the rectum of *Rhodnius* is responsible for water reabsorption. However, more recent work has more clearly defined the role of the rectum not only in water reabsorption, but also in the regulation of solutes. Several studies have shown that rectal fluid may be hypertonic to the haemolymph (e.g. *Schistocerca*, *Aedes*, *Rhodnius*, *Carausius*, *Tenebrio*, *Periplaneta* and *Calliphora*; see review by Kirschner[89]). However, the degree to which water and solutes may be subjected to reabsorption varies considerably. For example, larvae of the midge, *Aedes*, may produce fluid which is hypotonic to the haemolymph when the animals are in distilled water. When the larvae are in potassium chloride solutions, excess potassium is excreted. In sodium chloride solutions, excess sodium is excreted. Thus under a variety of experimental conditions the rectum of *Aedes* larvae is able to regulate the haemolymph. This ability is found also in the rectum of *Rhodnius* (Chapter 7). However, the powers of regulation of the haemolymph composition by the hindgut of *Carausius* appear to be limited.[165]

Phillips[144] has studied the function of the rectum of the desert locust, *Schistocerca gregaria* Forskål. He used a technique in which recta were isolated from the rest of the hindgut by ligation, leaving the tracheole and haemolymph supply intact. Various experimental solutions were introduced into the isolated recta and small samples were removed periodically for analysis. Movements of water between haemolymph and rectal lumen could be followed by measuring changes in the concentration of a non-reabsorbable solute, radioactive mammalian serum albumen, in the rectal fluid. Changes in the osmotic pressure and the concentrations of sodium, potassium and chloride in the rectal fluid were measured also.

The effect of the osmotic pressure of rectal fluid on the rates of water movement across the rectal wall in both directions was determined. Distilled water and hypoosmotic, hyperosmotic and isosmotic sugar (xylose) solutions were placed in the rectum. When an isosmotic (to the haemolymph) sugar solution was placed in the rectum, water was reabsorbed from it until the rectal contents were nearly dry. As shown in Fig. 30, there was net water movement out of the rectum except when the rectal contents were highly concentrated. The rate of water flow appeared to be approximately linear. When the osmotic gradient between the rectal lumen and haemolymph was *c.* 0·6 osmoles (rectum hyperosmotic to the haemolymph), no net water movement occurred. However, when the osmotic gradient exceeded 0·6 osmoles, there was net water movement into the rectal lumen.

The approximate linearity of the line in Fig. 30 suggested that superimposed on a passive water movement of 48 μl hr^{-1} per osmole of concentration gradient was water movement of 17 μl hr^{-1} due to some mechanism other than diffusion or hydrodynamic flow. This mechanism, although apparently not due to known passive forces, cannot be called active water transport, implying that a carrier of some kind is involved in moving water molecules. This non-passive water movement will be called 'activated' water movement here.

When the concentration gradient between the rectal lumen and the haemolymph was less than zero there was a passive water movement out of the rectum which was added to the 'activated' component to produce a large outward movement. When the gradient was greater than zero, there was passive diffusion of water into the rectum which could be subtracted from the 'activated' component. When the osmotic gradient between the rectal lumen and the haemolymph was 0·6 osmolar, the passive movement was equal to the 'activated' movement and no net water movement occurred (Fig. 30).

The haemolymph was diluted by feeding locusts on tapwater in water-saturated air, or concentrated by feeding them hypertonic saline in a dry atmosphere. Water reabsorption from hyperosmotic trehalose solutions placed in the rectum was then measured. Hydrated

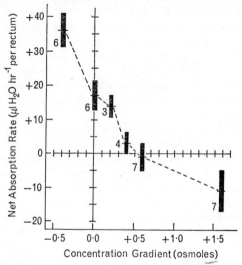

FIG. 30. Water movement in relation to the osmotic gradient in isolated recta of the desert locust, *Schistocerca*. From Phillips.[144]

locusts absorbed water from their recta less strongly than did dehydrated locusts (Table 16). These results demonstrated that the mechanism responsible for water reabsorption responds to a shortage or abundance of water by altering the rate of water reabsorption from the rectum.

Experiments were performed in which reabsorption of water from hyperosmotic saline by recta in hydrated and dehydrated locusts was measured. The results were quantitatively similar to experiments in which sugar solutions were placed in the recta. That is, water was reabsorbed in relation to the hydration state of the animal, not in relation to the ionic concentration of the rectal fluid. In these experiments, ions were reabsorbed with the water. Several alternative theories linking passive water movement with active processes were

TABLE 16

Freezing-point depression of the body fluids and the osmotic pressure gradient across the rectal wall of Schistocerca after the injection of a hyperosmotic trehalose solution into the rectum. From Phillips.[144]

	FREEZING-POINT DEPRESSION (°C)		
	Haemolymph	Rectal fluid	Gradient
	(a) Locusts fed on tap water		
Mean ± standard deviation	0·74 ± 0·06	1·30 ± 0·30	0·56 ± 0·26
	(b) Locusts fed on hyperosomotic saline		
Mean ± standard deviation	0·95 ± 0·07	2·74 ± 0·39	1·78 ± 0·40
Significance of difference between means (a) and (b)	significant	highly significant	highly significant

examined. None of these seem to apply to the rectum of *Schistocerca*. Therefore, Phillips proposed that water movement is due to some active process unknown in other fluid-transporting tissues.

The absorption of sodium, potassium and chloride from ligated recta was studied as follows: Sugar solutions which were hyperosmotic to the haemolymph were introduced into the recta. This prevented reabsorption of water. The solutions were made hypomolar or isomolar to the haemolymph with respect to the ions under study. In addition, measurements of the electrical potential across the rectal wall were made in normal and experimental animals.

There was a net reabsorption of ions from hyperosmotic sugar solutions whose ion concentrations were isomolar or hypomolar to the haemolymph. In both cases, the electrical potential difference (35 to 22 millivolts, lumen positive) suggested that chloride was actively transported. Absorption of sodium and potassium from isomolar solutions may have been passive. However, passive absorption of the cations from hypomolar rectal solutions would have required an electrical potential several times as great as that observed. These experiments indicated that under some conditions, at least, sodium, potassium and chloride reabsorption may be active.

Phillips studied the conditions under which rectal reabsorption of sodium, potassium and chloride could be saturated. In animals which were fed on tapwater and therefore had relatively low haemolymph ion concentrations, no saturation of the absorption mechanisms could be demonstrated. However, in saline-fed animals, in which the haemolymph was very much more concentrated than in tapwater-fed animals, saturation of the sodium, potassium and chloride absorption mechanisms was demonstrable. The rates of absorption of individual cations relative to rectal fluid concentration were measured. At any concentration of the rectal fluid, potassium was reabsorbed about ten times more rapidly than sodium. In further experiments, the nature of ion fluxes across the rectal wall was explored. From these experiments, and calculations based on the experiments, Phillips drew two main conclusions. First, the absorption of chloride by the rectal epithelium is clearly an active process. Secondly, sodium and potassium reabsorption probably involve an active component, but this could not be established unequivocally. The observed results are consistent with an hypothesis that absorption of water and ions is regulated by changes in the permeability of the rectal wall. Therefore, changes in the rate of transfer of ions, as observed in other epithelia, are not involved. Furthermore, this conclusion would appear to suggest that the rectal wall can differentiate between water and ions. Under conditions when it is absorbing ions maximally (water-fed locusts, low haemolymph concentration) water reabsorption is minimal. Conversely, when water is being reabsorbed maximally (saline-fed locusts, high haemolymph concentrations) ion reabsorption is not maximal. These results indicate that the rectum of *Schistocerca* is quite different from other fluid-transporting epithelia.

Measurements were made of the osmotic pressure and ion concentrations in the hindgut and rectum and the rate of flow of fluid into the hindgut from the Malpighian tubules. The locusts were fed on tapwater or hypertonic saline to lower or increase the haemolymph concentration. These measurements, together with the results of experiments on ligated recta, permitted an assessment to be made of the rôle of the renal system in osmoregulation. The results are summarized in Table 17.

In water-fed (hydrated) locusts, sodium, potassium and water from the Malpighian tubules flow into the rectum at a slower rate than they can be reabsorbed. Absorption of chloride may depend upon the nature

TABLE 17

Average rates at which substances flow into the rectum from the hindgut compared with their rate of absorption from the rectum, in Schistocerca. *From Phillips.*[144]

	Rate (μeq hr^{-1})			
	Na	K	Cl	H$_2$O
	(a) Locusts fed on tap water			
Inflow	0·16	1·11	0·74	440
Reabsorption	0·15	4·6	0·37*	935
	(b) Locusts fed on hyperosmotic saline			
Inflow	0·47	1·30	1·34	385
Reabsorption (max.)	0·38	0·72	0·38*	935 (?)

* Chloride reabsorption values relate to reabsorption from pure sodium chloride solutions and may not be typical of potassium chloride solutions.

of the cation with which it enters the rectum. In the presence of potassium it may be reabsorbed rapidly. Nevertheless, in water-fed locusts Malpighian tubule fluid is completely reabsorbed, yielding relatively dry excreta low in ions. In locusts fed on hypertonic saline a hypertonic fluid is retained in the rectum. The rate of entry of ions into the rectum exceeds the rate of reabsorption of ions, whilst water reabsorption continues. In fed animals the excreta normally present in the rectum cause loss of fluid and ions; these are retained in starved animals.

The selectivity to solutes of the rectum of *Schistocerca* may be due to the chitinous rectal intima. The permeability to water-soluble molecules of intimae isolated from recta and made into sacs was similar to the intimae in intact recta. Isolated intimae were impermeable to serum albumen and trehalose and permeable to smaller molecules. The water permeability of the cuticular intima was estimated to be about three times that of the exoskeleton.[146]

The function of the rectum of the blowfly, *Calliphora* was studied by Phillips,[145] using methods very similar to those described in studies of the locust. Artificial solutions were introduced into recta isolated from the rest of the hindgut by ligation. The blowflies were hydrated by feeding them on tapwater or dehydrated by denying them access to water. Chloride was not reabsorbed from artificial solutions injected into the recta of hydrated flies, but water was always absorbed. It was concluded that the rectum of *Calliphora* plays no part in ionic regulation during the production of haemolymph-hypoosmotic fluid, but it contributes to the production of an haemolymph-hyperosmotic rectal fluid by the reabsorption of water.

It has been suspected for some time that the rectal complex is responsible for the very dry faeces produced by the mealworm, *Tenebrio molitor* L. In a series of characteristically well-devised and patiently executed experiments, Ramsay and his colleagues[69,168] have provided evidence that this is so.

Faecal material enters the rectum of the mealworm suspended in fluid; most of the water is removed in the rectum prior to elimination of the faeces as pellets. Osmotic pressures and concentrations of sodium, potassium and chloride in the haemolymph and various spaces associated with the rectal complex (Fig. 29b) were compared. In general, the osmotic pressures of the anterior part of the perirectal space and the fluid in the Malpighian tubules were similar; in both spaces the osmotic pressure was usually well in excess of the osmotic pressure of the haemolymph. The osmotic pressure of fluid in the posterior part of the perirectal space was usually much greater than the osmotic pressure of the anterior perirectal space. There seemed therefore, to be an increasing osmotic gradient from anterior to posterior in the perirectal space; this probably paralleled a similar gradient in the adjacent Malpighian tubules. The osmotic pressures and ion concentration which may be achieved in the Malpighian tubules, perirectal space and haemolymph may be quite large by biological standards. The range of osmotic pressure of the Malpighian tubule fluid and perirectal space was from about 386 milliosmoles to about 4·3 osmoles. This is caused primarily by potassium chloride in the Malpighian tubule, but in the perirectal space, non-electrolyte of some kind contributes most of the osmotic pressure. The osmolarity of the haemolymph ranged from 386 to 754 milliosmoles. The higher osmotic pressures of haemolymph, Malpighian tubule fluid and perirectal space fluid were generally found in dehydrated animals.

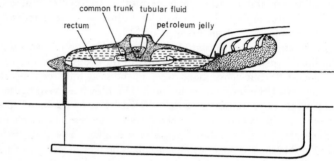

FIG. 31.   Technique for collecting fluid produced by the rectal complex of *Tenebrio* larvae. From Ramsay.[168]

Malpighian tubules were isolated in such a way (Fig. 31) that the rate of flow and osmotic pressure of fluid issuing from those parts of the tubules which are part of the rectal complex could be measured readily. Injection of distilled water and 3 molar sucrose into the rectum caused a rapid flow of fluid from the Malpighian tubules. The osmotic pressure of the tubule fluid decreased when 3 molar sucrose was injected into the rectum. However, there was no significant decrease in the osmotic pressure of the tubular fluid when distilled water was injected into the rectum. These experiments indicated that some of the water entering the rectum is removed by the Malpighian tubule component of the rectal complex.

When distilled water was injected into the perirectal space, fluid production by the Malpighian tubules increased rapidly. The osmotic pressure of the tubule fluid fell below that in the surrounding medium. Injection of 3 molar sucrose into the perirectal space created an abrupt cessation of fluid flow from the Malpighian tubules. This was considered to be due to 'damage' to the tubules.

Distilled water added to the medium surrounding the rectal complex had no appreciable effect on either Malpighian tubule fluid flow or tubule fluid osmotic pressure. Addition of 3 molar sucrose to the medium surrounding the rectal complex caused only a slight decline in tubule-fluid flow, but there was a marked rise in the tubule fluid osmotic pressure.

A decrease in the sodium : potassium ratio in the medium surrounding the rectal complex was followed by an increase in the rate of Malpighian tubule fluid flow and an increase in the osmotic pressure of the tubule fluid.

The foregoing experiments show conclusively that the rectal complex of *Tenebrio* is very permeable to water entering from the rectal lumen. However, they seem also to suggest that the perirectal Malpighian tubules are freely permeable to potassium. If this is so, then the potassium must pass from the haemolymph into the Malpighian tubule lumen without accompanying water; the osmotic gradient across the tubule wall is quite large, suggesting that the haemolymph and tubule lumen are not in functional contact with each other.

In further experiments[69] the permeability of the anterior and posterior parts of the rectal complex was studied. Radioactive sucrose and tritiated water were injected into the perirectal space. It was found that the anterior part of the rectal complex is much more permeable to both substances than the posterior part. Fluid in the posterior end of the perirectal parts of the Malpighian tubules has a higher osmotic pressure than does fluid in the anterior end. This parallels the osmotic pressure gradient seen in the perirectal space. Some hours after injection into the haemolymph, dye had accumulated in the posterior part of the perirectal space, suggesting that fluid moves in an antero-posterior direction in the perirectal space.

Rectal complexes were isolated in haemolymph or artificial media. These studies showed that both potassium and chloride are taken up by the rectal complex, but independently of each other. The electrical potential difference between the haemolymph and lumen of the Malpighian tubule part of the rectal complex averaged 48·5 millivolts (tubule lumen positive). This indicated that potassium is actively transported into the tubule but that chloride probably moves passively. It is most likely that this movement takes place through the leptophragmata, since those sites are most permeable.

Based on the results discussed above, Grimstone, Mullinger and Ramsay proposed a model to explain the function of the rectal complex in *Tenebrio* (particularly 'dry' animals). This model is illustrated in Fig. 32. The main input into the rectal complex is from the intestine. In the anterior part of the rectum fluid is rapidly reabsorbed, causing the suspended material in the intestinal fluid to be formed into faecal pellets. In the posterior end of the rectum air spaces surround the faecal pellets. Water is further removed from the faecal pellets in the posterior rectum by the absorption of water vapour by the rectal epithelium. The absorption of water as a vapour is probably active and is facilitated by the high osmotic pressure of the posterior part of the perirectal space. Some of the fluid absorbed in the anterior part of the rectum flows backward into the perirectal space. Water and sodium and potassium are taken up by

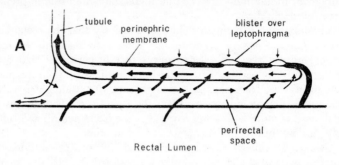

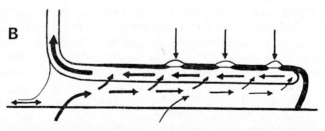

FIG. 32. Model of water (A) and potassium (B) movements in the rectal complex of *Tenebrio*. From Grimstone, Mullinger and Ramsay.[69]

the perirectal Malpighian tubules, resulting in an accumulation of non-electrolytes in the posterior perirectal space. Potassium is actively transported into the perirectal tubules via the leptophragmata, chloride flows passively. The leptophragmata cause potassium chloride to move into the rectal complex, but they 'resist' the tendency of water to follow. This creates the high osmotic pressure found in the posterior part of the rectal complex.

The rectal pad epithelia of the cockroach, *Periplaneta*, can vary the quality and quantity of the reabsorbed fluid in relation to the hydration state of the animal (Table 18). In normal animals, the fluid reabsorbed from the rectum is isosmotic to the haemolymph, since the rectal contents and haemolymph are isosmotic. In hydrated animals, the rectal contents are hypoosmotic to the haemolymph, indicating that a fluid hyperosmotic to the haemolymph is reabsorbed. In dehydrated animals the rectal content is hyperosmotic to the haemolymph indicating that the fluid reabsorbed is hypoosmotic to the haemolymph. In all cases, the potassium concentration in the rectal lumen was well in excess of the haemolymph potassium concentration; the sodium concentration in the rectal fluid was well below that of the haemolymph. These results indicated that sodium is reabsorbed from the rectal lumen in preference to potassium.

TABLE 18

Osmolalities of the haemolymph, rectal lumen contents and subepithelial sinus fluid of specimens of the American cockroach, Periplaneta, which were in a normal state of hydration or had been experimentally hydrated or dehydrated. Values are expressed as the mean plus or minus the standard error of the mean multiplied by two. From Wall and Oschman.[223]

	Normal	Dehydrated	Hydrated
Haemolymph	380± 4·1	436± 34·4	379± 4·5
Anterior lumen	409±77·4	572± 73·2	275±21·0
Posterior lumen	409±77·4	972±276	275±21·0
Anterior sinus	450±25·0	582± 62·8	363±18·8
Posterior sinus	460±14·2	620±149·6	391± 8·9

Like *Tenebrio*, *Periplaneta* appears to utilize extra-rectal spaces for fluid reabsorption. (Probably this is also true of other insects, but no direct studies have been made.) As shown in Table 18, the osmotic pressure of the subepithelial sinuses is always at variance with either the haemolymph or rectal-lumen contents. Furthermore, the sodium or potassium concentrations in the sinus fluids and haemolymph were always at variance. Wall and Oschman[223] have suggested that the haemolymph may not be the source of solutes in the subepithelial sinuses. They proposed a scheme of water and solute reabsorption from the rectum of *Periplaneta* based on the cycling of solutes within the epithelium of the rectal pads. This scheme is illustrated in Fig. 33.

Solute (sodium is illustrated) and water pass into the rectal epithelial cells which are assumed to be more concentrated than the rectal lumen. Solute is pumped into the narrow intercellular channels, making them very concentrated. Fluid from the intercellular channels flows into the intercellular spaces where it becomes diluted by the osmotic influx of water from the epithelial cell cytoplasm. The large intercellular spaces may become diluted to the same osmolality as the

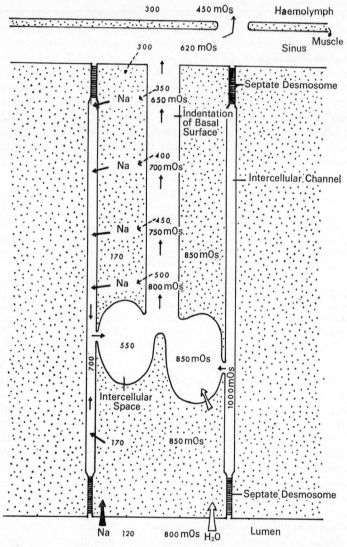

FIG. 33.   Rectal pads, with a proposed scheme for solute recycling. To illustrate how such a solute as sodium (Na) could be recycled, the concentration of sodium (plus anion, milliosmoles) that might be expected in various regions is given on the left in italics, and expected total osmolality (milliosmoles) is shown on the right. Bold faced values (lumen, sinus and haemolymph) are average determinations made on dehydrated animals. Other values indicated are highly spec-

cells, but solutes may still be more concentrated in the intercellular spaces than in the cell cytoplasm. The solutes could then diffuse down the concentration gradient into the cell, to be cycled back into the intercellular channels, *etc.* Fluid would be passed into the haemolymph via one-way valves in the muscle sheath overlying the epithelial sinus.

In the studies that have been considered thus far the major concern has been to demonstrate the function of the rectum in fluid water reabsorption. However, it may be recalled that the rectum of the mealworm may absorb water as water vapour. Recent studies on a thysanuran by Noble-Nesbitt[135] indicate that rectal reabsorption of water vapour may be a primary means of water balance. It was shown that when the rectal aperture ('anus') of the firebrat, *Thermobia domestica* (Packard) was blocked, uptake of water vapour from the atmosphere was halted. Many terrestrial arthropods appear to be capable of taking up water vapour from the atmosphere. It is possible that in these animals, in general, absorption of water vapour by the 'respiratory' surfaces or recta is important. As shown by the studies of Phillips and Dockrill,[146] the rectal surface of the desert locust may be about three times more permeable to water than is the body surface.

Studies of the fine-structure and function of insect recta show clearly that they are the reabsorptive part of the insect renal system. They appear to be peculiarly adapted to absorb fluid. However, despite fairly intensive study it is still far from clear how the rectal epithelia function. In Chapter 12 we shall consider some of the generalized models of fluid transport in living systems, and their possible applications to the insect rectum.

---

ulative, and are intended only as illustration. To generate a flow of water into the cell, it is presumed that the cell is more concentrated than the lumen. This may be accomplished by solute pumps located along the membrane facing the lumen. It is suggested that solutes are pumped into narrow intercellular channels so that the latter become quite concentrated. This fluid flows into larger intercellular spaces and becomes diluted, because of the osmotic influx of water from the cell. Large intercellular spaces may become diluted to the same total osmolality as the cell, but the concentration of transported solute (Na) would remain quite high relative to that in the cell. Solute could then diffuse down the concentration gradient back into the cell. This might occur (dashed arrows) as fluid flows along the indentations of the basal surface and perhaps also from the subepithelial sinus. Presumably the basal plasma membrane is relatively impermeable to water. Solutes may then enter narrow intercellular channels to be returned to the apical region, completing the cycle. From Wall and Oschman.[223]

Chapter 9

Renal function in Crustacea

Almost all knowledge of renal function in Crustacea derives from studies made on a few large decapods. Despite this the anatomy of decapod and non-decapod renal organs appears to be sufficiently similar to suggest that their basic functional characteristics will be similar. Known variations are probably related to habitat differences or to the relative degree of development of the different parts of the renal organs.

Structure of crustacean renal organs

Crustaceans, like other arthropods, possess two series of organs which may be classified as renal in function. These are the coelomoduct-derived maxillary glands and antennal glands, and the gut-derived rectal glands, cephalic glands and possibly, 'digestive' tubules.

Typically, the coelomoduct-derived renal organs consist of a coelom remnant, the 'coelomic' or 'end' sac, and a long tubule which opens to the exterior of the animal. In addition to the mesodermal component sometimes the extreme terminal portion is derived from an ectodermal invagination. Antennal glands open on the basal segment of the antennae, whilst maxillary glands open within the mouth parts. Often the tubule is dilated at its distal end, or empties into an urinary bladder.

In decapod crustaceans the simple form of the tubule becomes greatly modified, due to infolding and adhesion of the walls to form a labyrinthine structure. In freshwater crayfishes there is a long additional segment which superficially resembles a tubule (Fig. 34). However, the walls of this structure also are extensively infolded throughout most of its length. The location of the coelomoduct-derived renal organs varies from one group of crustaceans to another; it also varies within the same animal at different stages of the life cycle. For example, the maxillary gland is functional in the larvae of some decapods, whilst the antennal gland is the functional adult renal organ. Taking Crustacea as a whole, however, the maxillary gland is the commonest adult organ.[25]

The microscopical anatomy of antennal and maxillary glands of representatives of most crustacean groups has been studied, and descriptions are scattered widely in the literature stretching back in time for over a century. Here we shall confine our attention to electron microscope studies. Not only are they fewer in number, but the ultrastructure they reveal is more likely to have significance for functional comparisons and generalities.

The ultrastructure of antennal and maxillary glands

Electron microscope studies have been made of parts of the antennal glands of crayfishes,[1,3,93,131] all of the antennal gland of a crab, *Uca mordax*,[188] and the maxillary gland of the brine shrimp, *Artemia salina* (L.).[213-215] These studies highlight the uniformity of the structure of the coelomic sac in rather diverse crustaceans. However, they show also that the structure of the tubular parts of the coelomoduct-derived renal organs is diverse. Fig. 35 illustrates diagrammatically the kinds of cells known to occur in crustacean renal organs.

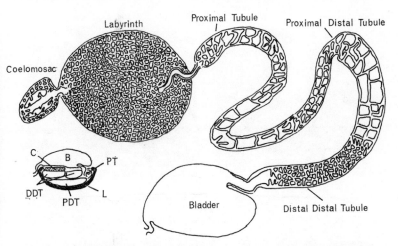

FIG. 34. *Large figure:* Antennal gland of the crayfish illustrating the relative size and extent of the parts. Also illustrated are the relative sizes of spaces within the organ. *Small figure:* Spatial relationships of parts in the intact antennal gland. *Abbreviations:* B = bladder, C = coelomosac, DDT = distal portion of the distal tubule, L = labyrinth, PT = proximal tubule and PDT = proximal portion of the distal tubule.

The cells of the coelomic (end) sac (Fig. 35a) are very similar to the podocytes of the vertebrate glomerulus (Frontispiece, lower photograph). They are not attached to each other at their lateral margins. Their bases rest upon the basement membrane by a series of interdigitating 'foot' processes. The gaps between the interdigitations of the foot processes (pedicels) are covered by a thin membrane. In the basal region of the cells may be seen invaginations of the cell membrane and small vesicles which suggest the occurrence of pinocytosis. The apical regions of the cells are filled with large, membrane-bound structures which have been called vacuoles or inclusions. When fixation is good,

E

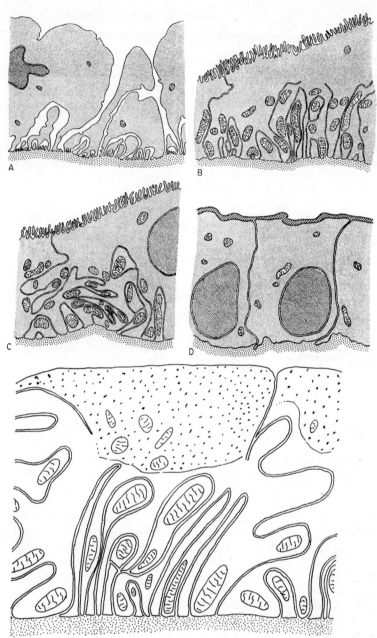

the membrane-bound structures are seen to have fixed arrays which appear crystalline, at least in *Artemia*[216] (Frontispiece, lower photograph). Mitochondria are few in number and scattered throughout the cell.

The cells of the proximal part of the efferent tubule in the maxillary gland of *Artemia* and the labyrinth of the antennal gland of the crayfish are shown in Fig. 35b. The cells vary in height and the junction between the lateral margins is simple. The basal membrane is infolded and mitochondria are enclosed within the folds. The mitochondria of the cells are generally associated with the lateral or basal cell membranes. Microvilli are present at the apical border of the cells. They are loosely arranged and in *Artemia* some of them are branched. The apical cytoplasm contains numerous small bodies which may be pinocytotic vesicles. In the labyrinth cells of the crayfish dense granules may be seen; these probably give that structure its green or yellow colour in life (hence the common name, 'green gland').

Figure 35c represents the appearance of cells in the distal part of the efferent tubule of the maxillary gland of *Artemia* and the labyrinth of the antennal gland of *Uca*. The cells have loosely-packed microvilli at their apical borders. The lateral and basal cell membranes are infolded in a complicated fashion, the folds enclosing mitochondria. The apical cytoplasm contains structures which may be pinocytotic vesicles. Superficially, at least, the cell type depicted in Fig. 35c looks like a mixture of the cell types depicted in Figs 35b and 35e.

Figure 35d represents cells from the terminal duct of the maxillary gland of *Artemia*. The only noteworthy feature of these cells is the presence of a cuticular layer which is probably continuous with the chitin of the exoskeleton of the animal. This part of the maxillary gland of *Artemia* is undoubtedly ectodermal in origin, not part of the original coelomoduct.

A cell 'typical' of the distal tubule of the antennal gland of the crayfish is illustrated in Fig. 35e. Here the basal membrane is elaborately infolded and large numbers of mitochondria are enclosed within the

---

FIG. 35. Ultrastructure of cells from various parts of crustacean renal organs, indicating the nature of cell borders and the numbers and distribution of cell inclusions. A. Podocytes of the coelomic sac. B. Proximal part of the efferent tubule of *Artemia* and the labyrinth of the crayfish. C. Distal part of the efferent tubule of *Artemia* and the labyrinth of *Uca*. D. Terminal duct of the efferent tubule of *Artemia*. E. Distal portion of the distal tubule of the crayfish. A, B, C and D supplied through the courtesy of Dr. Greta Tyson. E. Drawn from electron micrographs and description in Beams, Anderson and Press[3] and Miyawaki and Ukeshima.[131]

folds. The lateral membrane arrangements are very complicated; the membranes protrude far into neighboring cells. The apical membrane lacks microvilli; the cytoplasm of the apical part of the cell is undifferentiated except for a fine granular appearance. The fine structure of the proximal regions of the tubular part of the crayfish antennal gland has not been studied.

The function of decapod renal organs

The mechanism of primary urine formation

Studies of the vertebrate glomerular kidney have confirmed the view which saw the glomerulus as a filtration device. From that point on it became a simple matter, or so it seemed, to separate renal organs into two groups: 1) those which have a glomerulus or similar structure and 2) those which lack such a device. Kidneys in the first group are filtration kidneys; those in the second group, presumably, are secretion kidneys. As we shall see, once the functional characteristics of invertebrate renal organs became better known, it was discovered that matters are not quite so simple.

Investigations into the histological anatomy of renal organs revealed that the glomerulus is unique to vertebrates. It was clear that anatomical studies would not yield decisive evidence except in a few instances. Where there is no direct arterial supply to the renal organ, as in arthropod Malpighian tubules, there seems to be little likelihood that the filtration hypothesis applies. However, where an arterial supply to the renal organ was found (as in the higher Crustacea), it was possible that the filtration hypothesis would apply. Since anatomical criteria were inadequate bases upon which a final judgement could be made, there arose a series of studies in which physiological criteria were used to argue the pros and cons of the filtration hypothesis. The physiological criteria used were those derived from studies of glomerular kidneys. The pattern of excretion of a particular compound by an excretory organ under study was compared with the excretory pattern in the glomerular kidney. If the two patterns were similar, it was assumed that similar physiological processes were involved. If they were not similar, it was possible that filtration did not occur in the renal organ under study. For example, inulin is freely excreted by glomerular kidneys and not at all by aglomerular kidneys. On the assumption that inulin is filtered, then the invertebrate renal organs which excrete inulin are filtration kidneys.

Amongst the crustaceans the renal organs of only a few decapods have been studied in an attempt to determine whether or not physiological criteria for filtration exist. This evidence will be reviewed first and then its applicability to renal organs of lower crustaceans will be discussed briefly.

Answers to questions regarding the mechanism of primary urine formation of the antennal gland derive primarily from study of the freshwater crayfish. However, it is unlikely that the function of the antennal glands in other decapods differs in any significant way from the basic plan seen thus far in the crayfish.

As discussed in Chapter 2, glomerular filtration is thought to result from an excess of forces tending to push fluid into the nephron lumen over the forces tending to retain fluid within the blood space. Thus arterial pressure and the oncotic pressure of colloids in the primary urine tend to retain fluid within the lumen of the renal organ. The oncotic pressure of the blood plasma and hydrostatic resistance of the epithelia tend to retain fluid within the capillary space of the glomerulus.

Picken[147] measured the colloid osmotic pressure (COP) of the haemolymph and final urine, and the hydrostatic pressure of the haemocoel in the crayfish and shore crab, Carcinus maenas. In both he found that the haemocoelar pressure exceeded the haemolymph COP, which, in turn, exceeded the COP of the final urine. This indicated to him that filtration is possible in crustaceans. The validity of Picken's measurements may be questioned on several grounds, but these questions tend to show that his measurements of haemolymph COP were too high. Thus his main conclusion, that filtration is possible, would not be invalidated. Calculations of the probable COP of the haemolymph of crayfishes based on the amount of non-filterable protein (almost entirely haemocyanin of a molecular weight of c. 900 000) suggest that Picken's measurements were high by an order of magnitude.[90]

The excretion of polymers. Inulin is excreted freely by the antennal glands of all decapods into which it has been injected. As shown in Table 19, the inulin urine : haemolymph (U/H) ratio is not usually unity. This may indicate that some of the inulin is secreted, but the more likely explanation is that water is reabsorbed after formation of the primary urine. Binns[22] has argued that in animals which have extensive urinary bladders, such as crabs, inulin U/H greater than one may indicate a disequilibrium between the final urine concentration in the bladder and the concentration in the haemolymph. That is, it is presumed that the bladder has a large volume. The haemolymph inulin concentration falls steadily, whilst the bladder concentration falls more slowly. It is often seen, particularly in crabs, that the more rapid the rate of urine flow (i.e. the more rapidly the bladder is emptied) the lower the inulin U/H (cf. figures for 50% and 100% seawater in Table 19). However, this is almost certainly not the complete answer. Inulin U/H may exceed unity in macruran ('big-tailed') decapods,

TABLE 19

Inulin urine: haemolymph ratios (U/H) of decapod crustaceans under various experimental conditions.

Species	Experimental conditions	Inulin U/H	References and remarks
Crayfish	normal medium (freshwater)	2–3	90, 182
	normal medium (freshwater)	up to 28*	*antidiuretic due to handling[182]
	50% seawater	up to 31**	**antidiuretic[31]
Lobster (*Homarus americanus*)	normal medium (100% seawater)	1·0–1·1	32
Lobster (*Homarus vulgaris*)	normal medium (100% seawater)	1·17–1·51	31
Squat Lobster (*Galathea squamifera*)	normal medium (100% seawater)	1·21	30
Prawn (*Palaemon serratus*)	normal medium (100% seawater)	**1·75**	31
Fiddler crab (*Uca mordax*)	50%, 100%, 200% seawater	unity	188
Shore crab (*Hemigrapsus nudus*)	50% seawater*	0·92	*crabs remained immersed in the medium[183]
	100% seawater*	1·51	
	150% seawater*	1·33	
	50% seawater**	1·41	**crabs permitted to climb out of the medium[183]
	100% seawater**	1·22	
	150% seawater**	1·63	
Shore crab (*Carcinus maenas*)	50% seawater*	1·12	*crabs permitted to climb out of the medium[106]
	100% seawater*	1·51	
	150% seawater*	1·61	
	water-saturated air	2·5	
	100% seawater**	c. 2	*crabs permitted to climb out of the medium[183]
	50% seawater**		**crabs remained immersed in the medium[22]
	75% seawater**		
	100% seawater**	c. unity	

which have relatively small bladders. Furthermore, evidence from recent studies of both *Carcinus maenas* and *Portunus depurator*,[107] indicates that even in crabs appreciable water may be reabsorbed from the urine.

The only crustacean in which dextran excretion has been studied is the crayfish.[90] Like inulin, low molecular weight dextran (LMWD, mol. wt. = 15 000 to 20 000) and high molecular-weight dextran (HMWD, mol. wt. = 60 000–90 000) become concentrated in the final urine relative to the haemolymph. There is evidence that HMWD suffers restricted clearance by the antennal gland. Its clearance ratio (i.e. HMWD $U/H \div$ Inulin U/H) was 0·69, indicating that HMWD is cleared only about 70% as effectively as inulin. The antennal gland of the crayfish is more permeable to dextran than is the mammalian kidney (see Fig. 8 p. 33). Since HMWD is a range of polymers it would be expected that filtration would involve the selection of the smaller polymers in the range, as seen in dextran clearance studies on vertebrates.[73,225]

Blue Dextran 2000 is a dextran which has been conjugated to a blue dye. It is used as an easily visualized indicator to determine the void volume (space outside the gel) of columns used for gel chromatography. Rather surprisingly, Blue Dextran is excreted by the crayfish; at times in sufficient quantity to colour the urine pale blue-green (although the U/H is probably less than 0·1). Blue Dextran 2000 represents polymers whose molecular weights range from about 400 000 to 4 000 000. Nevertheless, it is excreted in the same range of molecular weights characteristic of the native material; there appears to be no selection for the smaller molecular weight polymers out of the range.[181] It has recently been discovered that Blue Dextran forms reversible complexes with various enzymes (e.g. yeast pyruvate kinase[72]). It is possible that Blue Dextran is secreted by the antennal gland after cellular uptake (see below p. 128).

Both the crayfish [*Pacifastacus leniusculus* (Dana)] and the lobster (*Homarus americanus* L.) excrete proteins in their final urine. Crayfishes excrete human serum albumin (MW $\simeq$ 70 000), but not mammalian (goat) serum globulin (MW $\simeq$ 180 000). The clearance of human serum albumin was restricted in that the U/H ratios averaged 0·50.[90] The lobster excretes dogfish (elasmobranch) plasma proteins and dogfish haemoglobin. The concentrations of the substances in the final urine relative to the haemolymph were not studied.[32]

The excretion of monosaccharides. Glucose excretion has been studied in a lobster, *Homarus americanus*,[32] several crayfishes[182] and the shore crabs, *Pachygrapsus crassipes* Randall[70] and *Carcinus maenas* L.[22] The glucose concentration in the urine is usually very low or nil. When sufficient glucose is injected into decapods to elevate the haemolymph levels above about 200 mg per 100 ml, glucose appears in the urine spontaneously.[22,32,182]

The glycoside, phlorizin, appears to block glucose reabsorption in the decapod antennal gland. When phlorizin is administered to crayfishes and to *Homarus* and *Carcinus*, glucose appears in the urine. In *Homarus* and *Carcinus*, the glucose U/H ratios approach unity. In crayfishes the glucose U/H ratios approach 2 to 3. That is, the glucose U/H during phlorizin poisoning tend to parallel the inulin U/H (Table 11), indicating that the appearance of glucose in the urine is due to failure in reabsorption.

The crayfish antennal gland apparently does not reabsorb the pentose, xylose, which appeared in the urine no matter what were the haemolymph xylose concentrations.[118] This result could be explained in two ways. First, xylose is not reabsorbed by the antennal gland, a result compatible with the results of studies of xylose excretion by the dog kidney (Chapter 5). Secondly, the result could be due to experimental design. During the experiments by Maluf[118] the nephropores of the crayfish were blocked prior to injection of xylose. Then, after the experimental period of some hours, all of the urine which had accumulated in the bladder was collected. The initial haemolymph xylose concentrations were well in excess of 200 mg per 100 ml, the approximate level which causes glucose to appear in the urine. It is possible that urine collected from the bladder at the completion of the experimental period contained xylose which had entered the urine during the time when the haemolymph xylose levels were very high[182].

At times, glucose may appear in the urine of decapods quite spontaneously, presumably due to stress. This effect is well known in vertebrates and is associated with elevated glucose levels in the blood (hyperglycaemia). In crayfishes glycosuria may be produced by excessive handling.[182] In the shore crab, *Carcinus*, glycosuria is seen in animals placed in dilute or poorly-aerated seawater[22].

There is little doubt that the coelomic sac of the antennal gland is the site of primary urine formation. Analysis of fluid within the coelomic sac should, therefore, give a clear indication of the process underlying primary urine formation. Such analyses have been made only in the antennal gland of the crayfish (Table 20). In the coelomosac, the concentrations of chloride, sodium and inulin are similar to those of the haemolymph, as is the osmotic pressure. These data indicate that the fluid in the coelomosac is derived from the haemolymph. However, the U/H for none of the above parameters is unity, as predicted by the filtration hypothesis. This could be due to a variety of reasons which have not been investigated so far, such as Donnan effects and electrical-potential differences. The concentration of potassium in coelomosac fluid is always well in excess of the potassium concentrations in the haemolymph. As will be discussed below, this may be due to secretion.

Reabsorption of solutes and water

It may be assumed that in antennal glands the primary urine is very like the haemolymph with respect to solute concentrations and osmotic pressure. Therefore, analyses of the final urine (or fluid within the various parts of the antennal gland) should reveal the extent to which the post-filtrational events are responsible for modifying the primary urine. The reader is referred to reviews of osmoregulation for details of reabsorption and secretion of ions.[104,154,189] Only those studies will be mentioned from which it is possible to derive information about mechanisms involved in reabsorption (and secretion).

Glucose. It is clear from studies, to which reference has been made above, that glucose is reabsorbed somewhere after its appearance in the primary urine. In crabs the site of reabsorption may be the bladder. Glucose is reabsorbed from solutions placed in the bladder of the shore crab, *Pachygrapsus crassipes*. The reabsorption is possibly blocked by phlorizin.[70]

The enzyme, alkaline phosphatase, has been localized histochemically at the lumenal borders of cells which transport glucose, and has also been localized in the cells of the labyrinth of the crayfish antennal gland.[90,116] However, it is by no means clear what relationship, if any, alkaline phosphatase bears to glucose reabsorption.[51]

Attempts to localize the segment of the crayfish antennal gland in which glucose is reabsorbed have failed. The compound 3-o-methyl-D-glucose was used. Methyl glucose is a compound whose chemical structure is altered in such a way that it cannot be metabolized. It is not reabsorbed by the vertebrate nephron from the urine. The antennal gland of the crayfish appears to be indifferent to it. Injected methyl glucose is readily reabsorbed by some tissue of the crayfish, but micropuncture studies have shown that its concentration in the antennal gland lumen is similar to that of inulin (Table 20).

Inorganic ions. The only ions which appear not to be reabsorbed by any part of the antennal glands of crustaceans are magnesium and sulphate (except in Mg-free seawater[107]). All other cations are reabsorbed to a greater or lesser extent. The most definitive information on the site of ion reabsorption may be derived from micropuncture studies of the crayfish antennal gland. Comparison of the U/H for sodium, chloride and inulin shows clearly that the two ions are reabsorbed in all parts of the antennal gland (Table 20). The U/H for sodium and chloride remain the same or fall whilst the inulin U/H rises. Since the osmotic pressure U/H remains close to unity, except in the distal tubule, it is likely that an isosmotic fluid is reabsorbed in all parts of the antennal gland. In the distal tubule, the chloride U/H falls precipitously, while the sodium U/H fall is less steep.

One of the interesting features of the micropuncture data shown in Table 20 is that they do not seem to confirm that the tubular part of the crayfish antennal gland functions to dilute the urine. However, this failure is only apparent. From the inulin U/H it may be seen that about 50 to 60% of the water in the primary urine is reabsorbed. At the same time, somewhat more of the sodium and chloride are reabsorbed, probably about 70 to 80%. Therefore, considerable solute is reabsorbed from the primary urine, much of it in the tubular portion of the antennal gland. The sodium and chloride concentrations of the fluid in the distal end of the distal tubule do not approach those of the final urine. Nevertheless, considerable dilution has occurred prior to the entry of the tubule fluid into the bladder. Final dilution of the urine must occur in the bladder, and there is experimental evidence in support of this.

Radio-active sodium placed in the bladder of the crayfish is transfered rapidly into the haemolymph. The transfer can be stopped by placing eserine in the bladder. Eserine inhibits the enzyme cholinesterase which is implicated in active transport of sodium in some tissues.[87]

There is evidence that in the crayfish, amino acids are also reabsorbed in the urinary bladder. The amino acid concentration in the distal part of the distal tubule is very high, but amino acids are absent from the final urine.[176]

Fluid

The excretory organs of crustaceans are probably important in fluid-volume regulation. When subjected to experimental conditions in which they tend to lose water across the surface of their bodies, some decapods react by increasing the reabsorption of water from their urine. This is illustrated in Table 19. The inulin U/H of animals kept in moist air or in concentrated seawater tend to be higher than in animals kept in more dilute seawater solutions.

Crayfishes and *Homarus* exhibit both osmotic and water diuresis. Diuresis results whenever fluid is injected into them, whether the fluid is hypotonic or hypertonic to the haemolymph.[32,172,180A] Injection of fluid into the crayfish causes the proximal part of the tubule to become most distended. This suggests that that part of the antennal gland is closely connected with water movements into the lumen.[180A] The

TABLE 20

Tubule fluid: haemolymph ratios (TF/H) of osmotic pressure and concentrations of sodium, potassium, chloride, inulin and 3-o-methyl glucose in various parts of the antennal gland of the crayfish. From Riegel.[180A] Differences between the average TF/H for osmotic pressure and sodium and potassium concentrations in summer (non-diuretic) and winter-spring (diuretic) crayfish whose means are shown in bold-face type, are statistically different at the 5% level of confidence.

Animal	Coelomosac	Labyrinth	Proximal Tubule	Proximal Distal Tubule	Distal Distal Tubule	Bladder
OSMOTIC PRESSURE TF/H						
Summer	1·03 ± 0·024	0·890 ± 0·017		0·830 ± 0·011	0·618 ± 0·028	**0·093 ± 0·002**
Winter–Spring	0·932 ± 0·051	0·997 ± 0·029	0·983 ± 0·043	0·927 ± 0·055	0·971 ± 0·046	**0·140 ± 0·023**
SODIUM TF/H						
Summer	**0·834 ± 0·035**	**0·831 ± 0·018**	0·773 ± 0·056	0·782 ± 0·061	0·755 ± 0·043	0·059 ± 0·006
Winter–Spring	**0·942 ± 0·032**	**0·926 ± 0·040**	0·911 ± 0·045	0·850 ± 0·046	0·720 ± 0·039	0·097 ± 0·028
POTASSIUM TF/H						
Summer	2·61 ± 0·413	**2·41 ± 0·322**	1·90 ± 0·126	**2·72 ± 0·449**	2·48 ± 0·311	**0·283 ± 0·101**
Winter–Spring	4·16 ± 0·687	**4·18 ± 0·766**	4·72 ± 0·813	**5·82 ± 1·03**	6·80 ± 0·849	**0·176 ± 0·036**
CHLORIDE TF/H						
	0·911 ± 0·018	0·886 ± 0·029		0·727 ± 0·075	0·454 ± 0·021	0·017 ± 0·004
INULIN TF/H						
	1·16 ± 0·061	1·35 ± 0·133	1·49 ± 0·186	2·12 ± 0·429	1·81 ± 0·250	1·60 ± 0·348
METHYL GLUCOSE TF/H						
	1·11 ± 0·138	1·34 ± 0·129	1·45 ± 0·165	1·68 ± 0·235	1·85 ± 0·245	1·19 ± 0·547

greatest concentration of inulin and un-reabsorbed solutes (e.g. potassium, Table 20, amino acids[180A]) is seen in the distal tubule of the crayfish. That portion is, therefore, likely to be a major site of water reabsorption in the antennal gland.

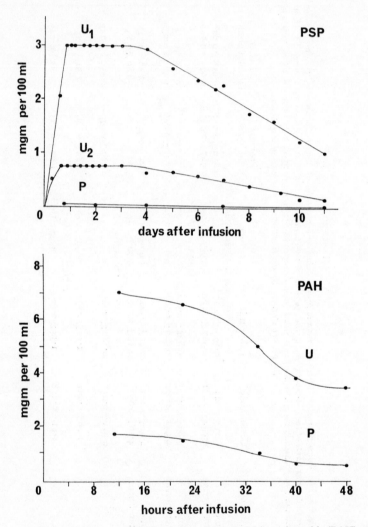

FIG. 36. Phenol red (PSP) and *para*-amino hippuric acid (PAH) secretion in the lobster, *Homarus americanus*. U = urine, P = plasma. From Burger.[32]

Secretion of urinary constituents

Numerous studies have been made of the secretion of dyes by the excretory organs of various crustaceans. Many dyes appear to be actively secreted because their concentration in the final urine is often many times the concentration in the haemolymph. The reader is referred to the reviews of Lison[101] and Maluf[118] for details and references to literature.

Phenol red (PSP) is secreted by both the antennal gland and the vertebrate kidney (Fig. 36). When the concentration of phenol red in the haemolymph is high, the U/P (U/H) ratio is at its lowest. However, when the haemolymph concentration falls, the U/P rises,[32] indicating that the dye enters the antennal gland by a saturatable transport mechanism. *Para*-amino hippuric acid is also secreted by the crustacean antennal gland (Fig. 36).[32]

Data in Table 20 indicate that potassium is secreted into the primary urine of crayfishes. There are two possible explanations for this. Potassium is associated with formed bodies which are secreted by the antennal gland (below p. 128). Secondly, potassium may be exchanged for another ion. As shown in Fig. 37, there is an inverse relationship between the sodium and potassium concentrations in the tubular part of the crayfish antennal gland. This may represent a sodium : potassium exchange mechanism as has been postulated for the glomerular nephron.[10]

Excretory organs of non-decapods

There is a remarkable similarity in the ultrastructure of the coelomic sacs of the decapods and the brine shrimp, *Artemia*, which should be reflected in a close functional similarity. If the structure of the coelomosac epithelium in decapods reflects the fact that filtration occurs there, then the same process should occur in the brine shrimp end sac. However, unlike decapods, the maxillary gland of the brine shrimp has no blood vessels leading directly to it. It 'floats' in the cephalic (head) haemocoel. Tyson[213,215] believes that arterial filtration is possible in the *Artemia* end sac despite the lack of an arterial supply. She has described connective-tissue strands which may hold open the lumen of the end sac. Furthermore, loops of the efferent tubule are fused by intercoil connexions which she believes may further increase the rigidity of the organ.

Formed bodies and crayfish renal function

Fluid removed from or produced by the antennal gland of the crayfish, the kidneys of frogs and some pulmonate gastropod molluscs and

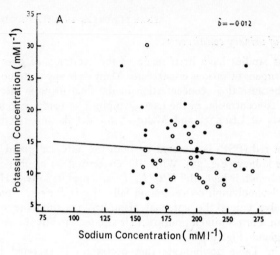

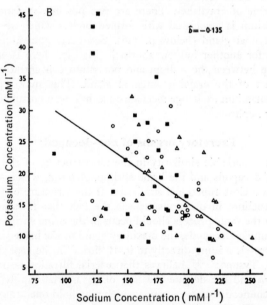

Fig. 37. *Upper figure*: Potassium concentrations plotted against sodium concentrations in the coelomosac (open circles) and labyrinth (closed circles). *Lower figure*: Potassium concentration plotted against sodium concentration in the proximal tubule (open circles), proximal distal tubule (open triangles) and distal distal tubule (closed squares). Note the inverse sodium : potassium relationship in the tubular parts. From Riegel.[177]

Malpighian tubules of insects contains formed bodies.[180A] The term 'formed body' is a collective designation for vesicular structures which exhibit a somewhat variable morphology. The formed bodies produced by the crayfish antennal gland have been studied most extensively and this review will be confined to a discussion of their structure and function.

Formed bodies appear to be produced by the cells of the coelomosac and labyrinth of the antennal gland. However, they may be seen in fluid removed by micropuncture from all parts of the antennal gland, except the bladder. Formed bodies produced by the coelomosac cells are spherical in shape with smooth boundary membranes. Accordingly, they have been called 'spheroids'.[175] They contain granules and smaller spheroids which vary in size from less than the resolving power of the light microscope ($< c.$ 0.3μ) to greater than 20μ. Formed bodies produced by the labyrinth cells are somewhat irregular in shape and have rough boundary membranes. They are called vesicles, and are generally in the order of 20μ in diameter. They also contain granules, vacuolated bodies and spheroids. Both spheroids and vesicles may contain multi-membranous structures.

The possible origin, function and fate of formed bodies

Electron micrographs of coelomosac cells reveal the existence of considerable pinocytotic activity, particularly in the basal region of the cells.[93] The apical cytoplasm of the cells is filled with membrane-bound bodies (see frontispiece). Kümmel[93] has suggested that the apical bodies arise by the fusion of smaller vesicles produced within the Golgi apparatus at the base of the cells. In size and general appearance the spheroids found in the lumen of the coelomosac resemble the apical membrane-bound bodies; it is likely that the former are those of the latter which have been released into the lumen. No detailed study has been made of the origin of the labyrinth vesicles; presumably a similar process is involved to that described for coelomosac spheroids.

As their primary function formed bodies probably play an important role in the elimination of surplus metabolites and foreign molecules. Dyes and dyed molecules appear to be incorporated into the formed bodies. For example, egg albumen which has been conjugated with Congo red may be seen in formed bodies. Similarly, when Congo red is injected into crayfish, it becomes conjugated with the haemolymph protein, haemocyanin. This process also dyes the formed bodies, particularly those produced by the coelomosac cells. In neither case can it be said with complete assurance that the Congo red which stains the formed bodies remains conjugated with the protein. However,

Blue Dextran 2000 is excreted intact by the crayfish antennal gland;[181] this compound can be seen to stain formed bodies in fluid samples removed from both the coelomosac and labyrinth. Cyanol, a dye which does not become conjugated with haemolymph proteins, is secreted by the cells of both the coelomosac and labyrinth. The blue dye can be seen to be retained within the formed bodies in micropuncture samples removed from the coelomosac and labyrinth. From the foregoing and other studies it may be surmised that formed bodies serve as a vehicle for the elimination of dyes and metabolites. However, it is now clear that their function is not limited to that of a carrier.

Formed bodies contain digestive enzymes which probably serve to hydrolyze molecules secreted within them.[175,176,180A] Quite possibly the accumulation of products of digestion within the formed bodies causes water to move into them osmotically, thus explaining why they appear swollen, especially in the distal parts of the antennal gland. The formed bodies probably burst after swelling to a critical size; normally they are not seen in bladder urine.

Fluid and solute movement due to the swelling of formed bodies.

Micropuncture samples removed from various parts of the antennal gland have been 'dialyzed' against crayfish-haemolymph-isotonic sucrose and Ringer. Dialysis consists of apposing a small droplet of micropuncture sample to a larger droplet of dialyzing solution. Separating the two droplets is a piece of filter whose pores are too small to permit formed bodies to pass. Therefore, the formed bodies are confined to the micropuncture droplet, but all dissolved solutes can pass freely between the two droplets.

The results of the dialyses revealed three events occurring concomitantly with the swelling of formed bodies. 1. Sodium and potassium are released from the formed bodies. Loss of sodium and potassium was most pronounced in ionic media (Ringer). Slightly acid Ringer caused sodium and potassium to be released in large amounts, whilst slightly alkaline media (Ringer and sucrose) retarded potassium loss. 2. Solutes in the fluid surrounding the formed bodies appeared to be excluded from them. This was true of lithium added to the dialyzing solutions and of sodium and potassium released from the formed bodies as they swelled. The foregoing effects are summarized and illustrated in Table 20A. The ratios of the concentrations of lithium, sodium and potassium in the micropuncture samples (C_{ms1}) and dialyzing solutions (C_{ds}) after dialysis are compared. 3. As the formed bodies in the micropuncture samples swelled during dialysis there was a movement of fluid into the micropuncture samples. In some cases (Table

TABLE 20A

*Summary of the ratios of the concentrations of
lithium, sodium and potassium in micropuncture
sample droplets (C_{ms1}) and dialyzing solution
droplets (C_{ds}) at the end of dialysis for 18 to 26 hours.
Data are expressed as the mean plus or minus the
standard error of the mean. Differences of the mean
C_{ms1}/C_{ds} ratios for sodium and potassium from the
mean C_{ms1}/C_{ds} ratios for lithium are statistically
significant (Probability greater than 99%) if the
mean is in bold-face type. Data from Riegel.*[179]

Li C_{ms1}/C_{ds}	Na C_{ms1}/C_{ds}	K C_{ms1}/C_{ds}
	SUCROSE DIALYSES	
0·776 ± 0·031	**1·02 ± 0·06**	**1·26 ± 0·11**
	ALKALINE RINGER DIALYSES	
0·816 ± 0·031	**0·881 ± 0·027**	**1·07 ± 0·06**
	ACID RINGER DIALYSES	
0·932 ± 0·015	0·922 ± 0·019	0·928 ± 0·018

TABLE 20B

*Net fluid movement into micropuncture samples dialyzed against sucrose and Ringer
solutions. Abbreviations:* DDT = *distal portion of the distal tubule;* LAB = *labyrinth;* COEL = *coelomosac. Data from Riegel.*[179]

Source of micropuncture Sample	Original volume (μl)	Net fluid movement (μl)	Dialyzing solution	Dialyzing Time (hours)
DDT	0·3	0·8	Sucrose	19
DDT	0·6	0·5	,,	22
DDT	0·2	0·1	,,	22
DDT	0·45	0·2	,,	22
DDT	0·6	0·3	,,	26
DDT	0·1	2·22	,,	17
DDT	0·24	3·54	,,	21
DDT	0·4	0·2	,,	5
DDT	0·4	3·7	Alkaline Ringer	24
DDT	0·36	0·85	,, ,,	5
DDT	0·36	0·55	,, ,,	5
LAB	0·35	0·3	,, ,,	20
COEL	0·35	0·1	,, ,,	21
DDT	0·18	0·35	Acid Ringer	19
COEL	0·13	0·8	,, ,,	3
LAB	0·16	0·65	,, ,,	3
LAB	0·05	0·42	,, ,,	3

20B) there was a net movement of fluid into the micropuncture
samples.

Based largely on studies of the behaviour of formed bodies *in vitro*
we may now summarize their characteristics. Formed bodies are pro-

duced by the cells of the coelomosac and labyrinth of the crayfish antennal gland as well as certain other renal organs.[180A] They may arise within cells by a process of pinocytosis. In their general form and possession of hydrolytic enzymes, some at least of the formed bodies are very similar to lysosomes.* When the formed bodies are released from the cells they swell and ultimately burst. As they swell, they release sodium (ionic media) and potassium (acid media). They appear to exclude solutes in the surrounding medium, possibly indicating that for a time they are permeable only to water. The possible importance of the characteristics of formed bodies to fluid and solute movements in the intact antennal gland will be discussed in Chaper 12.

* Unlike lysosomes, however, formed bodies are released from cells intact. Whether or not this is a genuine difference between formed bodies and lysosomes or merely reflects an ignorance of the ultimate fate of lysosomes remains to be seen.

Part 4: Renal Function in Other Invertebrates

Chapter 10

Renal function in molluscs, introduction

The reader is referred to the extensive review by Potts[153] for recent work not covered in detail here and for references to older literature. The molluscs have attracted considerable interest amongst invertebrate physiologists. As a consequence, some aspects of renal function have been studied in representatives of all of the major groups. Certainly, one of the attractions of the study of molluscs is their relatively large size; it is no accident that the molluscs whose excretory physiology is best known are very large.

The structure of molluscan kidneys

The renal organs of adult molluscs are modified coelomoducts. In most molluscs the coelomoducts lead from a coelom remnant, the pericardial space, to the outside of the animal or to the mantle cavity. The primitive function of the coelomoduct persists still in some molluscs, such as the ormer or abalone (*Haliotis*) where one pair of kidneys acts as a gonoduct additionally to its renal function.

There seems to be no single term which can be applied to the coelomoduct-derived renal organs of molluscs. In textbooks and the older literature, the term, 'nephridium', is sometimes used; such use is entirely inappropriate for adult molluscs. Here we shall use the functional term, 'kidney', following the usage of Potts.[153]

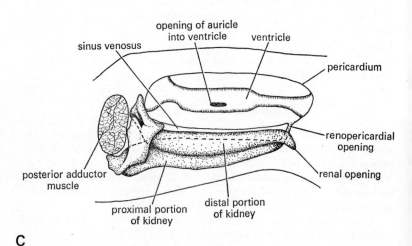

FIG. 38.   The arrangements of renal organs in molluscs. A, a primitive gastropod; B, a pulmonate gastropod; C, a lamellibranch; D, a dibranchiate cephalopod, *Octopus*. From Potts.[153]

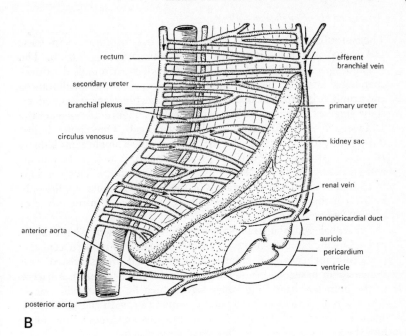

B

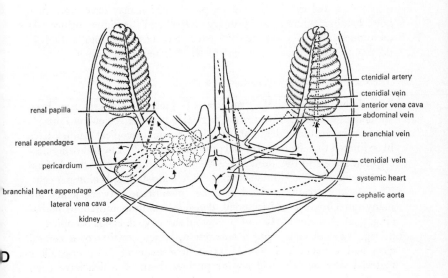

D

Arrangements of molluscan kidneys

The generalized arrangement of the kidneys in lamellibranchs (mussels and clams) and primitive gastropods is shown in Fig. 38a, b. The coelomic space is reduced to a pericardium which surrounds the three-chambered heart. Furthermore, the kidneys are paired. In lamellibranchs and primitive gastropods, one of the two kidneys functions as a gonoduct, conveying sex products to the mantle cavity. Figure 38c depicts the arrangement of the kidney in modern gastropods. One kidney is lost during the process of torsion so that there is only a single adult kidney. In some freshwater 'gilled' snails (prosobranchs), as well as the pulmonate snails, an ectodermal 'ureter' is added to the kidney. This develops from a groove in the mantle wall. The foregoing discussion applies only to adult molluscs, since true nephridia may be found in the larvae of some (Chapter 11).

In cephalopods the arrangement of the kidneys is somewhat complicated, but the basic elements are discernible still. In modern cephalopods (dibranchiates) the kidneys are paired and are associated with the lateral or branchial hearts which serve the gills (Fig. 38d). Adjacent to the branchial hearts are appendages which lie in coelomic spaces. The coelomic spaces or pericardia communicate with the kidneys by ciliated renopericardial canals, as in other molluscan kidneys. Protruding into the kidney sacs are so-called renal appendages.

In all groups of molluscs the basic elements of the coelomoduct are recognizable; a short duct leading from the coelom remnant (renopericardial canal), the kidney proper which may have more than one chamber (kidney sac, primary ureter) and the kidney orifice. As mentioned above, a secondary ureter may develop from a fold in the mantle wall which is not part of the original coelomoduct.

Microscopical anatomy of molluscan kidneys

The light-microscopical structure of mollusc kidneys has been studied extensively. The reader is referred to the review by Potts[153] for further details and literature. Electron-microscopical studies have been limited thus far to terrestrial pulmonates.[27,197] The following description relates to the kidney of *Achatina achatina*, one of the African giant snails.[197] The kidney sac epithelium consists of tall columnar cells. They have a greatly infolded basal cell membrane between which are many mitochondria and rounded, dense and multimembranous bodies (Fig. 39a). A major portion of the cytoplasm of each cell is occupied by a large vacuole containing a concretion, which consists of a central core and concentric layers of crystalline material. The crystalline material may be uric acid and/or purines, both of which have been found in the kidney of *Helix*. The apical border of the cells has well-defined microvilli, and the lateral borders between cells are relatively simple, except basally. The adjacent membranes are greatly folded basally (Fig. 39a).

The primary ureter of *Achatina* (Fig. 39b) is derived from the kidney sac and the cells superficially resemble those of the kidney sac. They lack the apical vacuoles and concretions, but there is a microvillous apical border. The lateral and basal cell membranes are extensively infolded and mitochondria are situated between the folds. Careful study of the arrangements of the membranes reveals that most of them are extensions of the lateral cell membranes. The cells are stellate in cross section (Fig. 39c), and they protrude extensively into neighbouring cells. The ultrastructures of the cells of the secondary ureter of *Achatina* are remarkably similar to those of the primary ureter.

Function of molluscan renal organs

Curiously, there is little anatomical evidence for a filtration site in any mollusc, yet no investigator of molluscan renal physiology seriously doubts that filtration occurs. The kidney lies adjacent to a source of high hydrostatic pressure, the heart. Even without the physiological evidence which we will review it would seem to be safe to surmise that filtration occurs in many molluscs.

Evidence for filtration

Pressure relationships. The circulatory system of molluscs, other than cephalopods, is classified as an open system. The haemocoels are not so extensive as in the arthropods and blood vessels are relatively well developed. The pressure requirements for filtration have been outlined in earlier chapters. A few measurements have been made of the blood (arterial) pressures and colloid osmotic pressure of mollusc blood. In the freshwater clam, *Anodonta cygnea*, the ventricular pressure averaged *c.* 6 cm H_2O and the blood colloid osmotic pressure (COP) averaged *c.* 0·4 cm H_2O.[148] In a freshwater pulmonate snail, *Lymnaea stagnalis*, the blood pressure was *c.* 8 cm H_2O and the blood COP averaged *c.* 0·4 cm H_2O.[148] The COP of the blood in the cephalopod *Octopus dolfleini* was 4 to 5 cm H_2O, whilst the blood pressure in the branchial heart may exceed that value by several times.[200] Therefore, in the few animals which have been studied, it appears that filtration due to blood hydrostatic pressure is possible.

A few studies of the effect of experimentally-altered blood pressures on the rate of pericardial fluid formation have been made. In the freshwater prosobranch snail, *Viviparus viviparus*, the rate of

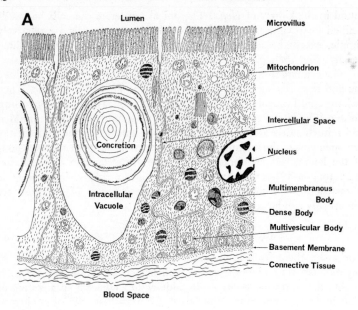

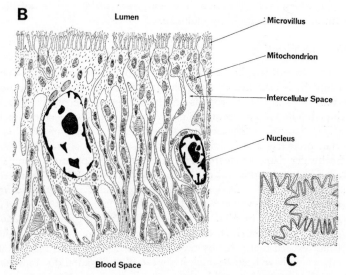

FIG. 39. Ultrastructure of cells typical of the kidney sac (**A**) and primary ureter (**B**) of *Achatina*. **C.** Way in which cells in the primary ureter interlock at their lateral borders. From drawings supplied through the courtesy of J. M. Skelding.

formation of pericardial fluid could be increased by increasing the
hydrostatic pressure of the blood.[103] Similarly, in *Octopus*, the rate of
formation of pericardial fluid was negligible when the blood pressure was
reduced to a level corresponding to the blood *COP*. Thereafter, the
rate of pericardial fluid formation was proportional to the blood pressure.[200] The rate of urine flow in the African giant snail, *Achatina
fulica* could be reduced to low levels by applying a back pressure to the
secondary ureter (Fig. 40). The inulin concentration of the urine
rose slightly, probably due to water reabsorption.[126] Similar results
were seen in experiments on *Octopus*.[124] The results described above

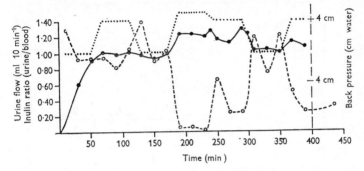

FIG. 40.   Effect of ureteral back pressure on the rate of urine flow and on
the inulin *U/B* in the kidney of *Achatina*. Open circles = rate of urine
flow; closed circles = inulin *U/B*; dotted line = ureteral backpressure.
From Martin, Stewart and Harrison.[126]

parallel those seen in studies of vertebrate kidneys. Augmentation of the
blood pressure in frogs leads to an increase in the formation of glomerular fluid.[171] Furthermore, production of a back pressure in the glomerular kidney by clamping the ureters leads to a diminution or cessation of
urine flow (see stop flow technique, Chapter 2).

The kidney sacs of molluscs are supplied with muscle fibres.[54] It
is likely that contraction of the muscles aids flow and mixing of the
kidney sac contents. In *Viviparus* the kidney sac alternately contracts
and expands. This action draws fluid out of the pericardium into the
kidney sac. It also ensures that the fluids come into intimate contact
with the cells of the kidney sac.[103]

Excretion of polymers and glucose. The freshwater clam, *Anodonta*
has a high concentration of protein and non-protein nitrogen in the
proximal part of the kidney sac (Table 21). Probably all molluscs may
be expected to have nitrogenous compounds in the kidney fluid. Fluid
in the kidney sac and primary ureter of *Achatina achatina* contains
formed bodies and crystalline material, which probably is uric acid.[196]

Inulin is excreted by a variety of molluscs: *Haliotis, Octopus*,[74] a prosobranch snail, *Viviparus*,[103] pulmonate snails, *Helix*,[196] *Achatina*,[126] a clam, *Anodonta*[151] and a mussel, *Mytilus*.[125] In all molluscs in which inulin clearance has been studied in detail (Part 4, p. 139), the inulin urine : blood ratio at the presumed site of filtration is close to unity. The clearance of small dextran molecules (16 000–19 000 molecular weight) by the kidney of *Achatina* is identical to the inulin clearance. However, larger dextran molecules (60 000–90 000 molecular weight) are cleared only about 65 to 70% as effectively as inulin.[196]

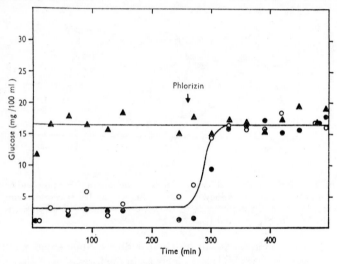

Fig. 41. Effect of phlorizin on glucose reabsorption from the pericardial fluid in the octopus. Triangles = blood glucose concentration; circles = pericardial fluid glucose concentration. From Harrison and Martin.[75]

Studies of *Haliotis, Achatina* and *Octopus* reveal that glucose is handled by molluscan kidneys in a manner very similar to the handling of that substance by the vertebrate kidney. The glucose concentration in the pericardial fluid of *Octopus* is normally quite low (Fig. 41). However, when phlorizin was added to the blood, the glucose U/B rose to unity. In *Achatina* the degree of absorption of glucose depended upon the rate of urine flow and the blood glucose concentration. At high rates of urine flow and high blood glucose concentrations (c. 200 mg per 100 ml) no absorption occurred. At low rates of urine flow and low blood glucose concentrations, reabsorption was greater than 90%. Phlorizin completely blocked glucose reabsorption in *Achatina*.

Site of filtration (a) *Physiological evidence.* Various studies have revealed physiological evidence for the filtration site in molluscan kidneys. Probably the least equivocal of these are the studies of Harrison and Martin[75] on *Octopus* and Skelding[196] on *Achatina*. In *Octopus* the renopericardial canal was ligated to prevent flow of fluid from pericardium to kidney sac of one of the kidneys. After ligation, no urine could be collected from the affected kidney sac. To simulate urine, the ligated kidney sac was filled with seawater. Inulin was injected into the animal and its concentration in the blood, pericardium on the ligated side and kidney sacs of both ligated and non-ligated sides were compared. The concentrations of inulin in blood, pericardium and unligated kidney sacs were approximately equal. Inulin failed to enter the kidney sac on the ligated side. This was fairly conclusive proof that the pericardium is the site of filtration in the octopus. Since most of the interior space of the pericardia of the branchial hearts of the octopus is filled by the branchial heart appendages, it is likely that filtration occurs from the branchial heart appendages.[75]

In some and perhaps all pulmonate gastropods the site of filtration appears to be the kidney sac. Only a small quantity (at most 0·1 ml) of fluid could be collected over several hours following catheterization of the pericardium of *Archachatina ventricosa* and *Helix pomatia*. By way of contrast, 15 to 50 times that quantity could be collected over a few hours following catheterization of the kidney sac.[219] Martin and his colleagues[126] were unable to collect fluid from a catheter inserted into the pericardium of *Achatina fulica*.

(b) *Morphological studies.* In a careful study of the ultrastructure of the kidney sac epithelium of *Achatina achatina*, Skelding[196] was unable to find an 'obvious' filtration site. All of the cells of the kidney sac are very similar in appearance to those depicted in Fig. 39a p. 136. Nevertheless, Skelding suggested that fluid moves across the epithelial cells possibly through extensive basal channels and apical microtubules. The large, iron-containing protein, ferritin (molecular radius = 55Å) was injected under pressure into blood vessels afferent to the kidney sac. Ferritin could be seen in the basal channels and apical tubules in electron micrographs of kidney sac cells of treated animals.

The actual filtration site in *Achatina* may be the basement membrane of the kidney sac epithelium. However, it is possible that preliminary filtration occurs from capillaries which ramify through the connective tissue overlying the kidney-sac epithelium. The dominant blood proteins of pulmonates are haemocyanins whose molecular weights may be several million. This protein is not seen in electron micrographs of the haemocoels which bathe the basement membrane of the kidney sac epithelium.

TABLE 21

Ratios of osmotic pressures and the concentrations of various solutes in the urine and blood of animals representing major molluscan groups.

ANODONTA CYGNEA (LAMELLIBRANCHIATA)

Measurement	Pericardium	Kidney Sac	Final Urine	References
Osmotic pressure	1·04*	1·16**	0·72**	*148 **49
Calcium	1·00	0·72	—	50
Chloride	1·00	0·56	—	50
Inorganic Phosphate	1·01	0·90	—	50
Protein Nitrogen	—	3·65	—	50
Non-protein Nitrogen	—	2·55	—	50

VIVIPARUS VIVIPARUS (GASTROPODA, PROSOBRANCHIATA)[1]

Measurement	Pericardium	Kidney Sac	Ureter	Urine
Osmotic pressure	0·95	0·36	—	0·19
Sodium	0·98	0·40	—	0·28
Calcium	0·81	0·43	—	0·26
Chloride	0·98	0·45	—	0·34

OCTOPUS DOLFLEINI (CEPHALOPODA, DIBRANCHIA)[2]

Measurement	Pericardium	Urine
Osmotic pressure	1·01	1·00
Sodium	1·01	0·98
Potassium	0·82	1·34
Calcium	0·94	0·53
Chloride	1·00	0·94
Sulphate	0·98	1·84

Table 21 *continued*

ACHATINA ACHATINA (GASTROPODA, PULMONATA)[3]

Measurement	Pericardium	Kidney Sac	Primary Ureter		Secondary Ureter	
			Proximal	Distal	Proximal	Distal
NORMALLY-HYDRATED ANIMALS						
Osmotic pressure	0·98	0·98	0·88	0·73	0·61	0·66
Sodium	1·04	1·00	0·93	0·73	0·60	0·30
Potassium	0·95	1·07	0·91	0·56	0·78	1·60
Calcium	0·62	0·65	0·53	0·36	0·23	0·22
Magnesium	0·90	0·94	0·88	0·68	0·92	1·21
Chloride	1·05	1·02	0·93	0·65	0·56	0·55
Inulin	1·02	1·03	1·12	1·32	1·38	1·50
DEHYDRATED ANIMALS[4]						
Osmotic pressure	0·98	0·99	0·77	0·60	0·46	0·64
Sodium	1·04	0·99	0·76	0·63	0·40	0·25
Potassium	0·95	1·15	1·05	0·74	1·16	2·44
Chloride	1·05	0·99	0·66	0·45	0·26	0·27
Inulin	1·12	1·12	1·63	1·89	2·12	3·12

1. Data from Little.[103]
2. Data from Potts and Todd.[155]
3. Data from Skelding.[196]
4. Dehydrated by ten per cent. of their body weight, including the shell.

The energy source for filtration in *Achatina* remains unknown. The kidney sac is well supplied with blood vessels, but these appear to be entirely venous.[196] The striking resemblance of the kidney sac cells to the cells of insect Malpighian tubules (cf. Figs. 39a and 19) suggests that filtration due to blood pressure may not be involved in primary urine formation in molluscs.

Analysis of fluid at the filtration site. The commonest site of filtration in non-pulmonate molluscs appears to be the coelom remnant, the pericardium. Evidence for this is seen in studies of gastropods, lamellibranchs and cephalopods. In cephalopods, the pericardia of the branchial hearts appear to be involved.

Table 21 summarized analyses that have been made of solutes and osmotic pressures in the blood, pericardium, kidney and final urine of various molluscs. The total osmotic pressure and the chloride, calcium and inorganic phosphate of the blood and pericardial fluid of *Anodonta* are identical. Furthermore, the protein content of the pericardial fluid is negligible. The fluid in the pericardium of *Octopus* and *Viviparus* and in the pericardium and kidney sac in the pulmonates is obviously derived from the blood. Although the pericardial fluid of *Achatina* is very similar to the blood, the pericardium is probably not the main site of filtration.

Post-filtrative events

In no case does the final urine of molluscs resemble blood in all respects and this is probably explained on the basis of post-filtrative secretion and reabsorption. There appears to be no Donnan effect between the blood and filtrate, which may indicate that the primary urine contains protein.

The final urine of marine molluscs is isosmotic to the blood.[153] In non-marine molluscs the situation may be otherwise; indicating some reabsorption in the kidney. In freshwater and terrestrial molluscs the urine may be isosmotic (*Theodoxus*[134]), slightly hypoosmotic (*Lymnaea*,[148] *Potamopyrgus*[210]), hypoosmotic (*Achatina*,[126] *Archachatina, Helix,*[219] *Anodonta*[148]) or markedly hypoosmotic (*Viviparus*[103]).

Reabsorption of solutes. Reabsorption of solutes, particularly ions, may be inferred from the observed osmotic pressures of kidney fluid and of urine shown in Table 21 and discussed above. In marine molluscs (*Octopus* and *Sepia*) there appears to be little reabsorption of ions. Sodium and chloride concentrations of the urine are less than those in the blood. However, the small differences observed may be due less to reabsorption than to replacement of these ions by ions which enter the urine after filtration. In non-marine molluscs there is clear-cut evidence for the reabsorption of ions. In *Anodonta* and *Viviparus*, both of which live in freshwater, all major ions (measured) are reabsorbed, and it is likely that this is the pattern in freshwater molluscs which produce significant quantities of urine. As discussed above, glucose is reabsorbed in all molluscs in which its excretion has been studied.

The most exhaustive and definitive study of the function of a mollusc kidney has been made by Skelding[196] on the African giant snail, *Achatina achatina*. Average osmotic pressures and concentrations of solutes in filtrates of micropuncture samples are shown in Table 21 as ratios of the osmotic pressures and concentrations of solutes in filtered blood samples. Studies were made of normally-hydrated and partially-dehydrated animals. Hydrated animals were actively feeding and crawling about in a moist atmosphere. Dehydrated animals were kept in a dry atmosphere, which caused them to retreat into their shells and lose about ten per cent. of their body weight.

In normally-hydrated specimens of *Achatina* about one-third of the water and solutes are reabsorbed by the time the primary urine leaves the secondary ureter. The preponderance of this reabsorption occurs in the primary ureter; the reabsorbed fluid is hyperosmotic to the plasma. This is indicated by a fall in the osmotic pressure U/B ratio in the primary ureter. One of the consequences of dehydration is an increase in the reabsorption of water from the primary urine, as might be expected. However, at the same time, hyperosmotic fluid reabsorption in the primary and secondary ureters is intensified.

Secretion of solutes. Sulphate appears to be secreted by *Octopus* (Table 21) in common with most marine animals. Hydrogen ion appears to be secreted in the kidneys of *Viviparus* and *Octopus*, in which the final urine is more acid than the primary urine. The pH of the pericardial fluid in *Octopus* and the urine in the secondary ureter of *Archachatina* and *Helix* are more alkaline than the blood.[219] Whether this is due to secretion of bicarbonate or phosphate or reabsorption of hydrogen ion (or, indeed, quite another process) cannot be ascertained.

As shown in Table 21, both potassium and magnesium are secreted into the urine of *Achatina achatina;* secretion of these ions is most marked in the secondary ureter.

A large variety of organic substances appear to be secreted in Molluscs. As shown in Table 21, protein appears to be secreted into the kidney sac of *Anodonta*. This is true also of 'non-protein nitrogen', the nature of which remains unknown.[50] *Para*-amino hippuric acid (PAH) and phenol red are secreted by the kidneys of molluscs. There is good evidence that the pathway of secretion is identical for the two compounds as in the vertebrate kidney. They compete with each other and their excretion is affected by the same metabolic inhibitors. The

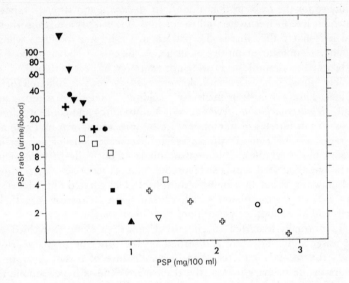

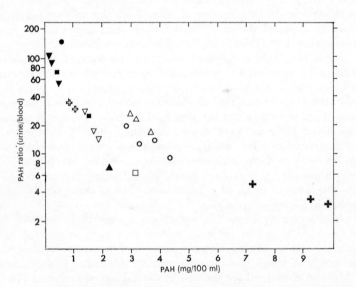

FIG. 42.   Urine : blood ratios for phenol red (upper figure) and *para*-amino hippuric acid (lower figure) in relation to the blood concentrations of those substances in the octopus. From Harrison and Martin.[75]

two compounds are secreted by the kidneys of *Haliotis*[74] and *Achatina*.[126] The most exhaustive study of PAH and PSP excretion in molluscs is that done on *Octopus*.[75] When the blood concentrations of PAH and PSP were low, the urine concentrations were high (Fig. 42). The fall of the PAH and PSP U/B when the blood concentration of either substance is elevated suggests that a transport mechanism became saturated. When both PAH and PSP were perfused into the blood, the excretion rate of both substances was lowered, suggesting competitive inhibition. The inhibitor, 2,4-dinitrophenol affected the excretion of both compounds; the secretion mechanism may depend upon oxidative phosphorylation. Further, the inhibitor, Benemid, inhibited PAH and PSP secretion. Benemid inhibits the organic acid secretory pathway in the vertebrate kidney, probably competitively.

The abilities of kidneys of molluscs to concentrate PAH may be compared. The maximum concentration (i.e. PAH U/B) by *Haliotis* was about 5, and *Achatina* seems less able than *Haliotis* to concentrate PAH. By way of contrast, the octopus achieved a maximum urine concentration of PAH some 155 times that in the blood. This value compares favourably with the concentration of PAH by the mammalian kidney. For example, in man, the PAH U/B ratio may reach 260, but this is due primarily to the reabsorption of water. The clearance ratio (PAH $U/B \div$ inulin U/B) in man reaches a maximum of about 5. In the octopus the maximum PAH clearance ratio was about 150. Therefore, secretion may play a relatively more important rôle in the excretory processes of the octopus than it does in man.[75]

Nitrogen compounds of various kinds are major constituents of molluscan kidneys and urine. However, the mechanics of nitrogen excretion has been afforded scant attention beyond the cataloguing of the various nitrogen compounds found in kidneys and the possible significance of their presence. The reader is referred to Potts[153] for a recent review of the subject and for references.

The study of Potts[152] on ammonia excretion in *Octopus* is of a type which should form the basis of other studies. The concentration of ammonium in the urine of the octopus is proportional to the concentration of hydrogen ion (Fig. 43). In effect, the more acid is the urine, the greater is the concentration of ammonium relative to the blood. As discussed in Chapter 2, it is thought that ammonia is trapped in vertebrate kidneys as an ion, after diffusing into the lumen of the nephron as dissolved gas. Potts suggested that the same mechanism exists in the octopus kidney. The octopus excretes an acid urine (pH $\simeq$ 5) which has a high ammonia concentration.

To increase the ammonia concentration of the blood, small quantities of ammonium chloride were injected into octopi. The blood, pericardial

F

fluid and kidney sac fluid were then analyzed for pH and ammonia concentration. Table 22 shows a result typical of the experiments. The blood of the octopus was normally weakly alkaline or weakly acid (i.e. average pH $\simeq$ 7). [By way of contrast, the pericardial fluid was normally more alkaline and the kidney sac fluid was normally

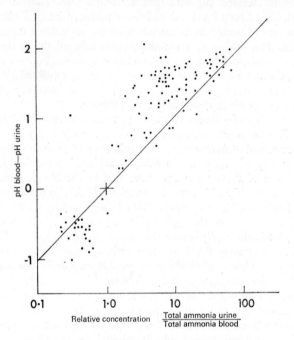

FIG. 43. Concentration of ammonia in the urine relative to the concentration of ammonia in the blood compared with the difference between the pH of the blood and urine in the octopus. The lower the pH of the urine, the higher is the ammonia concentration in the urine. From Potts.[152]

more acid than the blood. The concentrations of ammonium in the three fluids were found to be proportional to the acidity of the fluids (Table 22). In further experiments the kidney sacs were irrigated with acid and alkaline buffered seawater. Again, the ammonia concentration in the kidney sac was proportional to the acidity of the introduced solutions.

As discussed in Chapter 5, acidification of the urine in vertebrates is caused by the entry of hydrogen ion into the lumen; at least some of the hydrogen ions are derived from the ionization of carbonic acid in the cells (presumably). Production of carbonic acid in the cells is due to the action of the enzyme, carbonic anhydrase, which accelerates the hydration of carbon dioxide. This reaction can be blocked by the inhibitor substance, Diamox, which prevents or diminishes acidification of the urine. However, a different mechanism of acidification of the urine may be present in the octopus kidney. Urine acidification was unaffected by Diamox.[152]

Reabsorption of water. The kidneys of molluscs are capable of water reabsorption; this is seen most clearly in gastropods. Vorwohl[219]

TABLE 22

Ammonia concentration and pH of the blood, pericardial fluid and kidney sac fluid in an octopus, after injection of 1 ml of 0·5 molar ammonium chloride at 1·5 hours (arrow). From Potts.[152]

Time (hours)	Blood	pH Kidney sac	Pericardium
1	7·12	6·00	7·82
→			
2	7·09	—	7·82
3	7·02	5·56	7·61
4	7·01	5·50	7·57
5	7·02	5·40	7·62

Time (hours)	Blood	Ammonia (mM l⁻¹) Kidney sac	Pericardium
1	0·16	13·5	0·09
→			
2	1·36	—	0·61
3	—	30·0	0·27
4	0·60	24·0	0·22
5	0·34	18·0	0·19

perfused saline through the ureters of the pulmonates *Helix* and *Archachatina*. The final volume collected at the distal end of the ureters was only about 77% (*Helix*) and 60% (*Archachatina*) of the initial volume. Similar experiments done on specimens of *Viviparus* by Little[103] showed that about 25% of the perfusate was reabsorbed. However, further experiments on *Viviparus* indicate that greater water reabsorption is possible in the unperfused kidney. As shown in Fig. 44, the inulin U/B in fluid issuing from the kidney sac may exceed two. Thus more than 50% of the water in the urine may be reabsorbed before the presumptive urine enters the ureter in *Viviparus*. Similarly, in *Achatina*, the inulin U/B of ureter fluid varies inversely with the rate of urine flow. At high rates of urine flow (80–170 μl min^{-1}) the inulin U/B approximated unity. At low rates of urine flow (10–80 μl min^{-1}), the inulin U/B rose to values in excess of two.[126] These values for inulin U/B were obtained by catheterization of the kidney during which free flow of fluid occurred. It is doubtful if free-flow exists in the uncatheterized animal. The secondary ureter of *Achatina* possesses a muscular wall which probably prevents this. As shown in Table 21, in the uncatheterized animal, inulin U/B over three occur when the snails are partially dehydrated.

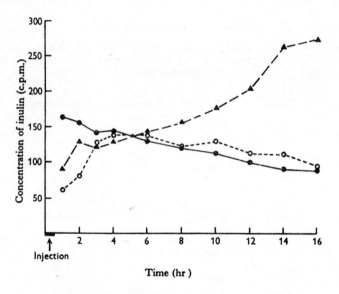

FIG. 44. Concentration of inulin in the blood (closed circles), pericardial fluid (open circles) and initial (pre-ureteral) urine (triangles) in *Viviparus*. After Little.[103]

Chapter 11

This chapter will be concerned with a sampling of a large assemblage of animals about whose renal function little is known. These include annelids, protozoans and 'miscellaneous' animals. By 'miscellaneous' is meant a few representatives from the groups which possess protonephridia.

Renal function in annelids

Annelids differ from the invertebrate groups discussed so far in that they possess an extensive coelom and a closed circulatory system. Thus there are two distinct extracellular fluid compartments, the coelomic fluid and the blood.

As discussed in Chapter one, the renal organs of metazoan animals are derived from coelomoducts or nephridia (as well as the gut). Adult animals of the groups discussed previously utilized coelomoducts or gut appendages as their renal organs. In annelids, the renal organs are nephridia or mixtures of nephridia and coelomoducts (nephromixia). Nephromixia are widespread in the polychaetous annelids, but in the other classes of the phylum, generally, the renal organs are nephridia.

The structure of annelid renal organs

The metanephridia of two annelids, *Lumbricus terrestris* L. and *Hirudo medicinalis* L. will be considered here. *Lumbricus* is an earthworm belonging to the class Oligochaeta; *Hirudo* is a member of the class Hirudinea, the leeches. Whilst these two species may not be considered as representative of the phylum Annelida or even of their respective classes, they are the only annelids whose excretory organs have been studied in any definitive way. The reader is referred to the reviews of Goodrich[62] and Bahl[2] for extensive surveys of the morphology of annelid renal organs. Books by Laverack[96] and Mann[119] and the review by Oglesby[135A] give details of excretion in annelids which are not discussed here.

The structure of the metanephridium of Lumbricus. The nephridia of *Lumbricus* are large; they open to the coelom proximally, and distally they open to the outside of the body. As shown in Fig. 45a, the nephridium of the earthworm is highly differentiated and forms three major loops. The parts of the nephridium which comprise the first two loops are embedded in a mass of cortical cells (indicated by black in Fig. 45a) or intercellular substance. Ramifying through the cortical-cell mass are blood vessels. All three loops of the nephridium are enclosed in a membrane made up of coelomic (peritioneal) cells.

Graszynski[68] has made a study of the fine structure of the nephridium of *Lumbricus*. The cells which border the nephridial canal are highly differentiated. The distribution of cilia and microvilli at the apical borders of the nephridial cells is shown in Fig. 45b. Also shown in that figure is the occurrence and general development of basal infoldings. Aside from the variations illustrated in Fig. 45b, the cells of the individual parts of the nephridia vary considerably in height. Within individual nephridial parts the cell height may measure from two to three microns to about 15 μ. The cytoplasmic inclusions include mitochondria which may be scattered in the cytoplasm or localized between the basal infoldings. The extensive description of Graszynski[68] should be consulted for further details.

Graszynski paid particular attention to two previously-expressed contentions, firstly, that the lumen of the nephridial canal is intracellular, and secondly, that filtration could occur across the walls of the blood capillaries into the tubule lumen.[2] The cells of the various parts of the nephridial canal are generally flat and very wide. This is indicated by the observation that nuclei and lateral cell borders are only infrequently observed. Nevertheless, the appearance of the borders of the cells left Graszynski with the impression that the lumen of the canal is intercellular, not intracellular, as supposed previously. Bahl[2] suggested that filtration could occur from the blood capillaries to the lumen of

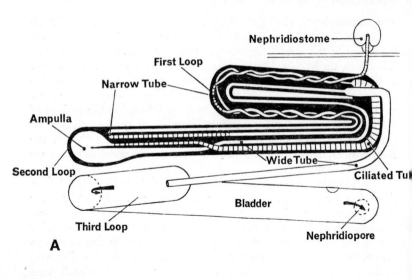

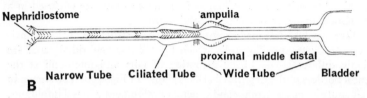

FIG. 45. A. Gross anatomy (very diagrammatic) of the earthworm nephridium. B. Distribution of microvilli, cilia, and basal infoldings in various parts of the nephridium of the earthworm. From Graszynski.[68]

the nephridial canal. However, in *Lumbricus* the blood vessels do not border on the lumenal epithelium. There is at least one layer of cells between the epithelium of the blood vessels and the epithelium of the canal. This makes it unlikely that filtration could occur directly from the blood vessels into the lumen of the nephridial canal.[68]

Function of nephridium of Lumbricus

The function of the nephridia of only two species of earthworms has been studied in any detail. These are *Lumbricus* and *Pheretima posthuma*. Bahl's study[2] indicates that *Pheretima* produces a very dilute final urine, but it provides few clues as to other processes of urine formation such as the site and possible mode of formation of the primary urine. Studies of *Lumbricus* have utilized the direct micropuncture approach, so it is possible to interpret results more easily. Therefore, further remarks will be confined to studies of *Lumbricus*.

As shown in Table 23, urine collected from the nephridiopore of *Lumbricus* is markedly hypotonic to the body fluids. It seems reasonable to assume that this is due to the activity of the nephridia. The function of the nephridia consists of the conservation of solutes and the elimination of water. The obvious source of primary urine in open nephridia is the coelomic fluid. The blood and the coelomic fluid are very similar in composition (Table 23); it is possible that the coelomic fluid arises from the blood by filtration, but the location of the filtration site has

TABLE 23

Comparison of the ion concentrations and osmotic pressure in blood, coelomic fluid and final urine of Lumbricus *kept in tap water. Data under columns headed '1' from Kamemoto, Spalding and Keister.*[88] *Data in columns headed '2' from Ramsay.*[159]

Measurement	Blood	Coelomic fluid		Urine
	1	1	2	2
Sodium (mM 1^{-1})	83·6	78·1	—	—
Potassium (mM 1^{-1})	5·3	2·7	—	—
Calcium (mM 1^{-1})	6·1	2·3	—	—
Chloride (mM 1^{-1})	47·2	48·5	46·2	3·4
Osmotic pressure (= mM 1^{-1} NaCl)	*	*	90·6	17·1

* Blood osmotic pressure averaged 9·7 mM 1^{-1} less than the coelomic fluid in 27 of 31 earthworms kept in tapwater, moist soil or saline. In the remainder, the osmotic pressures of the blood and coelomic fluid were identical.[159]

not been investigated. Whatever its origin, it seems likely that the coelomic fluid serves as the primary urine in *Lumbricus* and perhaps other oligochaets which possess open nephridia. Coelomic fluid may move into the preseptal portion of the narrow tube by the action of the cilia of the nephridiostome. These cilia may act also in selecting out the large coelomic fluid cells.

Micropuncture studies of the concentrations of chloride and the osmotic pressure of fluid in the nephridium of *Lumbricus* are summarized in Fig. 46. The fluid in the most proximal part of the nephridium, the narrow tube, is isosmotic with the bathing medium. In the middle tube there is a slight fall in the osmotic pressure, but the greatest dilution occurs in the wide tube, particularly in the distal part. Therefore,

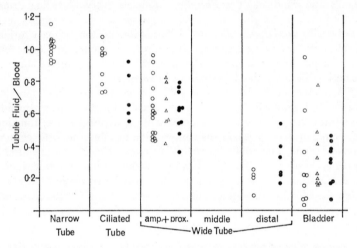

FIG. 46. Osmotic pressures (open circles = Ramsay's daa;[160]t open triangles = Boroffka's data) and chloride concentrations (closed circles) in various parts of the nephridium of the earthworm. From Boroffka.[23]

micropuncture studies indicate that a fluid very similar to the coelomic fluid enters the nephridiostome (or proximal part) of the nephridium. This fluid then is altered by reabsorption of solutes, producing a hypotonic final urine.

Boroffka[23] has extended the stopped-flow microperfusion technique developed on vertebrate nephrons to studies of *Lumbricus*. She injected test solutions containing sodium chloride and/or mannitol into the proximal part of the wide tube. The solutions were isosmotic to the bathing solution. Sodium and chloride were reabsorbed from the perfusion solutions containing those ions (Fig. 47). However, the equilibrium concentrations were higher than during free-flow conditions, i.e. test solutions perfused into the wide tube were not diluted as much as is the fluid normally found there. When isosmotic mannitol was perfused, sodium and chloride moved into the perfusate. At equilibrium, the concentrations of sodium and chloride corresponded closely to the concentrations of those ions found in the tubule lumen under free-flow conditions. This suggested that some non-reabsorbable solute must be present in the tubule fluid to promote maximum sodium and chloride reabsorption. The microperfused volumes of the solutions of mannitol and sodium chloride remained constant. This indicated that water was not reabsorbed from the proximal part of the wide tube under the conditions of microperfusion.

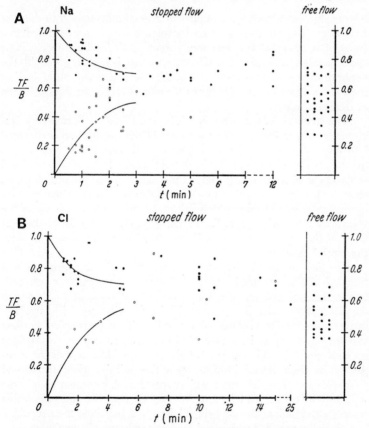

FIG. 47.   Stopped-flow microperfusion studies of the proximal portion of the wide tube in the earthworm nephridium, compared with free-flow micropuncture. The proximal portion of the wide tube was perfused with isosmotic mannitol (open circles) or isosmotic saline (closed circles). From Boroffka.[23]

Boroffka also measured the transcellular and transtubular electrical potential differences in order to establish if transport of sodium and chloride is active. Under stopped-flow conditions the net transtubular electrical potential difference averaged 11 millivolts (lumen negative). The calculated active transport potentials (Nernst equation) for sodium and chloride were, respectively, -20 and -3 millivolts. Therefore, it was concluded that sodium is actively transported against the electrochemical gradient, whilst chloride moves passively.

Structure and function of the nephridium of the medicinal leech, Hirudo

The nephridia of leeches are similar in general morphology to those of *Lumbricus*. They possess a ciliated structure which is suspended in a sinusoid remnant of the coelomic space; in all leeches the coelomic space is greatly reduced. The ciliated structure is homologous with the nephridiostome of oligochaets.[62] In *Hirudo* and many other leeches there is no communication between the ciliated structure and the lumen of the nephridium.

The structure of the metanephridium of *Hirudo* is shown very diagrammatically in Fig. 48. The main body of the nephridium is disposed into four lobes, the initial, apical, inner and main lobes. The central (nephridial) canal is found within all but the initial lobe. From proximal to distal the central canal is divided into five regions: the initial, inner, short, wide (proximal and distal) and end canals. The end canal empties into an extensive bladder which in turn empties to the exterior of the animal by a nephridiopore. Ramifying through the matrix of the four lobes of the nephridium are small canaliculi which communicate with the central canal.

Boroffka and her colleagues[24] have studied the fine structure and function of the metanephridium of *Hirudo*, with particular reference to the site and manner of primary urine formation. The cells which surround the canaliculi (the nephridial lobe cells) are fairly uniform in their ultrastructure. They possess microvilli at their apical borders and the basal region is extensively infolded. Between the basal folds are mitochondria which are found also in the middle area of the cytoplasm. At their lateral borders, near the apical region, the lateral membranes of the cells are very close together. A basement membrane separates the nephridial lobe cells from the connective tissue cells which comprise the bulk of the nephridial lobes. The matrix of the nephridial lobes is richly supplied with blood capillaries whose walls are fenestrated.

In order to discern the pathway of fluid flow in the nephridium, Ringer containing the dye, lissamine green was injected into the canaliculi and central canal in various parts of the nephridium. The flow of

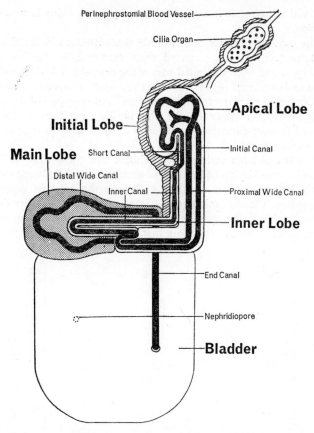

FIG. 48. Nephridium (very diagrammatic) of the medicinal leech, *Hirudo*. From Boroffka, Altner and Haupt.[24]

fluid was then observed with a stereomicroscope. The most probable course of fluid flow within the nephridium was from the canaliculi of the initial lobe to the canaliculi of the main lobe, inner lobe and apical lobe, thence into the central canal opening within the apical lobe.

The foregoing study established that fluid flow probably originates in the extensive canalicular system of the nephridium. In order to obtain evidence of the mechanism of primary urine formation, inulin was injected into the dorsal blood vessel. Urine was then collected by catheterization of the nephridiopore and analyzed for inulin. In only two samples (of 13) was there any but a negligible amount of inulin in the final urine. It was concluded that inulin does not normally enter the urine and therefore it is unlikely that the primary urine is formed by filtration.

The osmotic pressure and chloride concentrations in blood and in micropuncture samples removed from canaliculi in the inner and apical lobes and from the initial part of the central canal were analyzed. These analyses (Fig. 49) showed that the osmotic concentrations of the blood and fluid removed from the canaliculi and early part of the central canal are similar. However, the chloride concentration of the fluid removed from the canaliculi and central canal was greatly elevated compared to the blood.

Boroffka and her colleagues concluded that the primary urine in *Hirudo* is formed by both filtration and secretion. Fluid is filtered through the pores in the blood capillary walls into the adjacent connective tissue spaces. Electron micrographs failed to reveal sites where fluid in the connective tissue space may have free access to the canalicular lumen. It was assumed therefore that the movement of fluid from the

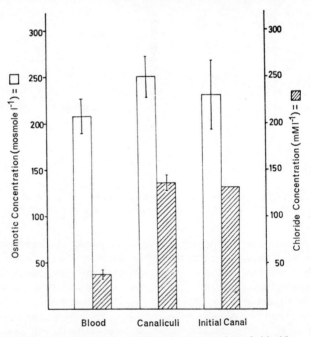

FIG. 49.   Osmotic pressure and concentration of chloride of the blood compared to fluid removed from the canaliculi of the inner and apical lobes (canaliculi) and the initial part of the central canal (initial canal) of *Hirudo*. From Boroffka, Altner and Haupt.[24]

connective tissue space to the lumena of the canaliculi was due to secretion. This may explain why inulin does not enter the urine in appreciable quantities. It was suggested that fluid secretion in the nephridium of *Hirudo* may be due to active solute transport.

Excretion in animals possessing protonephridia

Protonephridia are closed renal organs, consisting of simple or multiple tubules, each of which ends in a single terminal cell. The terminal cell may possess a tuft of cilia (flame cell, Fig. 50a) or a long flagellum, (solenocyte, Fig. 50b).

Protonephridia are the commonest of the renal organs in invertebrates. They are found principally in the acoelomate phyla (Platyhelminthes, Rotifera, Nemertinea, Acanthocephala, Priapulida, Entoprocta, Gasterotricha and Echinodera). They are found also in adult coelomates

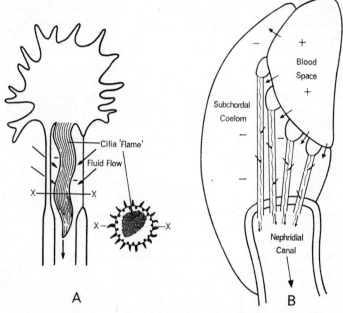

FIG. 50. A. 'Flame' cell (cyrtocyte) from the protonephridium of the miricidium larva of a liver fluke. *Small diagram*: Transverse section taken at X—X on the cyrtocyte. B. Diagram of cyrtopodocytes in the protonephridium of *Branchiostoma*. In A and B, positive and negative signs indicate areas of possible high and low pressure, respectively; arrows indicate the possible sites and direction of fluid flow. From Kümmel.[94]

(Annelida: Polychaeta and Archiannelida; Cephalochordata) as well as larval coelomates (Annelida: Polychaeta and Archiannelida; Echiuroidea, Mollusca, Phoronida, Cephalochordata).

Until recently it has been possible only to infer from structure what the functional mechanism of the protonephridia may be. It has been considered that the beat of the 'flame' or flagellum of the terminal cell sets up a 'negative' pressure within the tube. This suction then draws fluid across the thin membrane of the neck of the terminal cell.[124]

Fine structure of the terminal cells of protonephridia

The terminal cells are the most proximal part of the protonephridia to the body cavity. Therefore, interest has been created by the possibility that a knowledge of their fine structure will provide evidence for the mechanism of primary urine formation. The structure of the flame cell of the miricidium larva of the liver fluke (*Fasciola*) will serve as an illustration. As shown in Fig. 50a, the flame cell consists of a cell body from which strands of cytoplasm radiate. The cell is continued as a hollow tube (barrel) within which is found a ciliated tuft. As shown schematically in Fig. 50a, the barrel of the flame cell is composed of alternating rods which are separated by a boundary membrane. This arrangement suggests a barrel and the name 'cyrtocyte' ('barrel-flagella cell') has been applied to it.[94] Between the inner and outer rods of the 'barrel' there are small interstices or slits which are about 100 Å in diameter. The slits are covered by the boundary membrane.

The fine structure outlined above has been seen in the protonephridia of several animals: a turbellarian flatworm (*Stenostomum*); another trematode, *Schistosoma*; a priapulid, *Halicryptus*; the entoprocts, *Urnatella* and *Pedicellina*; the rotifer, *Asplanchna*; a gastrotrich, *Chaetonotus*, and a polychaet annelid, *Glycera*. A variation on the above-described arrangement of rods and boundary membrane has been noted in the protonephridium of the larvae of the gastropod mollusc, *Lymnaea*. The boundary membrane appears to be absent; instead there is a basement (fibrillar) membrane which envelops the whole barrel. The structure of the boundary membrane is quite different from the structure of the basement membrane and is suggestive of a unit membrane. In the entoprocts and priapulids which have been studied, the basement membrane is present in addition to a distinct boundary membrane.

The structure of the protonephridia of the cephalochordate, *Branchiostoma* (formerly *Amphioxus*) appears to be more specialized than the structure of protonephridia of other invertebrates (Fig. 50b). The terminal cells (cyrtocytes) rest against a blood space; the barrel (tube) penetrates through the subchordal coelomic space to protrude into the head of the nephric tubule. The barrel is composed of ten three-cornered rods and it is not bounded by any membrane. Within the barrel lies a single flagellum. The blood space lacks an endothelial lining; instead it is enclosed by a basement membrane which appears to be a product of the cell bodies of the cyrtocytes. This arrangement bears a resemblance to the podocytes of vertebrates and crustaceans. For this reason, the terminal cells have been called 'cyrtopodocytes' by Kümmel.[94]

Function of the terminal cells

Knowledge of the fine structure of the terminal part of the protonephridia permits a number of inferences to be made as to the function of that part. In the protonephridia of most invertebrates fluid may gain access to the nephridial canal only after passing through a membrane surrounding the barrel of the terminal cell or cyrtocyte. It is possible that the major source of energy in all but, perhaps, *Branchiostoma* is the beat of the cilia or flagella.[94] It has been argued[34] that the suction created by the beat of the flame would be insufficient to overcome the colloid osmotic pressure of the tissue fluids. Ciliated chambers of sponges, isolated under cover slips, could generate a pressure of only a few millimetres of water. However, as correctly argued by Pantin,[141] it is doubtful if these measurements have relevance to terminal cells. The cross-sectional diameter of the flagellated chambers of sponges is very large (1 mm or larger) and the suction generated within them is dissipated over a large surface. On the other hand, the cross-sectional area of the barrel of the flame cells is small (less than 5μ). Suction generated by the beat of the flame would be dissipated less readily.

The cyrtopodocytes of *Branchiostoma* may represent a situation more readily comparable to that seen in the flagellated chambers of sponges. The site of application of the pressure head may have been transferred from the barrel of the terminal cell to the membrane surrounding the blood space. Thus fluid may be forced to move from the blood space into the relatively large subchordal coelom. Under these conditions, the suction created by the beat of the flagellum in the terminal cell may be augmented by blood pressure (Fig. 50b).

Despite fairly extensive knowledge of the structure of protonephridia, few functional studies have been made. The only obvious reason for this is their small size. Pantin[141] observed oscillations of the tube wall in the flame cells of the terrestrial nemertean, *Geonemertes*. These oscillations indicated that the tube wall responds to pressure changes, but they failed to indicate clearly the source of the pressure. Danielli and Pantin[40] localized the enzyme alkaline phosphatase in the canal part of the protonephridia of *Geonemertes* and a turbellarian flatworm, *Rhynchoderis*. This enzyme is implicated in a number of active-transport processes. Its absence from the terminal cells of the protonephridia suggested that those structures do not serve a role of active transport.

Pontin[150a] has observed that in the large rotifer, *Asplanchna*, parasitic bacteria which are seen occasionally in the body space (pseudocoel) are drawn toward the terminal cells of the protonephridia. Braun and his colleagues[29] suggested that this could have been caused either by suction created by the beat of the ciliated tuft of the terminal cells or by turgor pressure caused by movements of the animal's body. Warner[226] has published indirect experimental evidence that the beat of the ciliated tuft in the terminal cells of *Asplanchna brightwelli* is responsible for movement of fluid into the protonephridium. The effect of pressure in the pseudocoel was eliminated either by puncturing the integument of the experimental animals or isolating the protonephridia in drops of body fluid. In either case, the rate of urine formation (indicated by the rate of pulsation of the bladder) was diminished, but is was not halted completely.

Some indirect experimental studies indicate that filtration underlies primary urine formation in protonephridia. Further, they show that the protonephridia may have reabsorptive powers.

The protonephridia of *Asplanchna* empty into a contractile bladder, which empties to the exterior by the ureterovesical duct. Urine was collected from the ureterovesical duct of animals isolated on microscope slides under liquid paraffin. A micropipette was inserted into the opening of the ureterovesical duct and fluid expelled during several contractions of the bladder was collected.

The osmotic pressure and the concentrations of sodium and potassium in the urine were considerably less than the osmotic pressure and concentrations of ions in the body fluid (Table 24). Conservation of solute, especially sodium, was marked when the animals were trans-

TABLE 24

Concentrations of sodium, potassium and inulin and the osmotic pressure of body fluids and urine of rotifers, expressed as urine: body fluid ratios. The rotifers were specimens of Asplancha priodonta *kept in habitat water or distilled water. From Braun, Kümmel and Mangos.*[29]

	Lake water	Distilled water
Osmotic pressure U/BF	0·52	0·23
Sodium U/BF	0·64	0·23
Potassium U/BF	0·39	0·34
Inulin U/BF	1·42	—

ferred from habitat water (lake water) to distilled water. Most significantly, inulin was freely cleared by the protonephridium of the rotifer.
This result strongly supported the contention that the primary urine is
formed by filtration. The fact that the urine : body fluid ratio for inulin
was greater than unity and that the U/BF for sodium, potassium and
osmotic pressure are less than unity, indicates that post-filtrative
reabsorption occurs. Thus, despite a morphology which is 'different',
the protonephridium seems to function like other filtration kidneys.

That the protonephridium of the rotifer is able to alter its function
in response to environmental alterations is shown in Table 24. Furthermore, as calculated by Braun and his colleagues, the urinary loss of
sodium in distilled water was only about 40% of the loss in the normal
medium, although the output of urine is slightly greater in distilled
water than in habitat water.

Excretion in Protozoa

The mystery of the contractile vacuole of the Protozoa has occupied
morphologists and physiologists for many years. The small size of the
contractile vacuole (at most a few microns in diameter) has thus far
frustrated extensive direct study. As a consequence, the current concepts
of the functional mechanism of the structure has been arrived at by a
process of the elimination of untenable theories.

Fine structure of the contractile vacuole

The contractile vacuole may be a permanent or temporary organelle
within the cytoplasm of the protozoan cell. In general, in amoebae, they
tend to be temporary, and do not appear to occupy a fixed position.
In ciliates and flagellates they are fixed both in structure and location.
Several studies have been made of the ultra-structure of contractile
vacuoles. These have revealed details of the differentiation of the
cytoplasm surrounding the vacuole. The reader is referred to the
review by Kitching[91] for a much more detailed treatment of structure
and function than can be given here.

The contractile vacuole of *Amoeba* is bounded by a double unit
membrane. Just outside the membrane is a zone filled with small
vacuoles and outside this zone is a ring of mitochondria. The fixed
contractile vacuole of *Paramecium* (Ciliata), Fig. 51, has quite a different
structure from that of amoebae. It is fed by a series of canals which
radiate from the vacuole proper. As the vacuole fills, the canals become
dilated and fluid is forced into the contractile vacuole. Study of the
ultrastructure of the contractile vacuole apparatus of *Paramecium
caudatum*[192] has revealed a complex structure. As shown in Fig. 51,

the radial (uriniferous) canals run through a region of the cytoplasm filled with a network of fine tubules (uriniferous tubules). Distal to the uriniferous canal, the uriniferous tubules communicate with the endoplasmic reticulum. The uriniferous tubules communicate with the radial canal, but only while that structure is expanding. Expansion of the radial canals occurs whilst the contractile vacuole proper is contracting; see Fig. 51a. The proximal ends of the radial canals expand distally to form ampullae which lead into injector canals and thence to the contractile vacuole proper. Contraction of the radial canals and vacuole proper may be brought about by the contraction of fibres (Fig. 51) found in their walls.

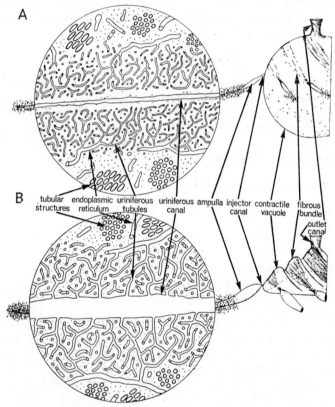

FIG. 51.   Fine structure of the contractile vacuole and one uriniferous (radial) canal in *Paramecium*. A. Vacuole full, uriniferous canal not in communication with the uriniferous tubules. B. Vacuole filling, uriniferous canal in communication with the uriniferous tubules. From Schneider.[192]

The foregoing describes the two main variations of the contractile vacuole apparatus in protozoans. However, much more information is available and the reader is referred to reference 91 for further details.

Function of the contractile vacuole

As the result of recent ultrastructural studies, contractile vacuole function is better understood as a morphological phenomenon. However, we are only a little more enlightened as to the functional relationships in the vacuole.

The role of the contractile vacuole is probably mainly osmoregulatory. If this is true, clues to its functional mechanism may be had from the effects on its function of alterations in the osmotic environment of the protozoans. The contractile vacuole is a fairly constant feature of freshwater Protozoa, whilst it may be absent in marine and endoparasitic protozoans. This suggests at once that its role is osmoregulatory; perhaps functioning to rid the body of osmotic water. Rhizopod (amoebae) and ciliate protozoans have been transferred from freshwater into various concentrations of seawater. In general, the rate of pulsation of the contractile vacuole (= vacular output) varied inversely with the concentration of the medium.[91,157] This implies that the osmotic pressure of the protozoan cell in freshwater exceeds that of the medium, and several indirect studies confirm this. The cell volume of freshwater Protozoa diminishes in solutions of non-electrolytes whose concentrations are greater than about 50 to 80 milliosmoles. This possibly indicates that the cytoplasm of freshwater protozoans has an osmotic pressure equal to 50–80 milliosmoles. However, the difficulties inherent in accepting values derived from such studies may be seen from a comparison of two such studies on *Amoeba proteus*. Mast and Fowler[129] found that specimens of that species shrank in non-electrolyte solutions whose concentrations were 5 mM l^{-1} or greater. However, Schmidt-Nielsen and Schrauger[191] made direct measurements of the melting-point depression of cytoplasm samples removed from specimens of *A. proteus* by micropuncture. These indicated that the cytoplasm has a concentration averaging 101 milliosmoles.

It is probably true that the internal concentration of freshwater protozoans is well in excess of the concentration of their medium. A few studies have shown that the contribution of metabolic water and water taken up by the food vacuoles is negligible relative to the osmotic uptake of water. However, in marine protozoans, uptake of water in the food vacuoles may account for the amount of water put out by the contractile vacuoles, this amount being much reduced from that estimated to be put out by the contractile vacuoles of freshwater protozoans. Therefore, in freshwater Protozoa, the contractile vacuole may function to remove osmotic water, whilst in marine protozoans, the contractile vacuole may function to remove water released by metabolism.

In a direct study of the contractile vacuole, Schmidt-Nielsen and Schrauger[191] demonstrated that the contractile vacuole fluid of *Amoeba proteus* has an average concentration of 32 milliosmoles. This compares with concentrations of the cytoplasm and medium of 101 and 8 milliosmoles, respectively. These studies provide little direct evidence for the mechanism of vacuole formation except to show that it is probably an active process. Various studies have shown that the metabolism of protozoans must be intact for vacuole formation to continue normally. Anoxia, cyanide poisoning and high hydrostatic pressures all halt or depress vacuolar activity. It is probable that these effects arise from the deprivation of an energy source for vacuole formation.[91]

Part 5: Some Theoretical Considerations of Fluid Movement

Chapter 12

Introduction

It should be clear from the preceding chapters that renal organs exist to generate a flow of fluid. The common and highly generalized view of the function of this fluid flow is 'to rid the body of wastes'. In general accounts, sight is often lost of processes which are equally if not more important than ridding the body of wastes. One of these processes is fluid volume control. When faced with an excess body water load animals respond by producing urine very rapidly (diuresis). In the process they may lose large amounts of solutes. However, the solutes can be recovered from extra-renal sources. The renal organs appear to control the overall fluid balance of the body.

In this chapter we shall explore some of the ways that fluid flow in renal organs is initiated and controlled. This discussion has been deferred to the last chapter because, like trying to explain to a virgin the joys of making love, it is difficult to explain fluid movement prior to extensive exposure to moving fluids.

The nature of water movement

Water has a structure derived from electrostatic interactions between its molecules, called hydrogen bonds. The hydrogen bonds impose limitations on the movement of individual water molecules. When the energy of water molecules is increased part of the extra energy is utilized to disrupt hydrogen bonds.

Water molecules can be made to move in a directional sense in two or possibly three practicable ways. First, water may move down a kinetic energy gradient established by osmotic pressure. In this case, water will move away from a place where it is more concentrated toward a place where it is less concentrated. Second, water may move down a kinetic energy gradient established by hydrostatic pressure. In this case, the concentration of the water may not vary, but the kinetic activity of the molecules may be increased due to a restriction upon the volume which can be occupied by water and other molecules. Finally, water may move by active transport up an energy gradient. To accomplish this, the water molecules may be 'bound' to some kind of carrier resulting in a diminution of their energy.

In most instances of water movement in biological systems, it is considered that water moves down a kinetic gradient established by differences in osmotic or hydrostatic pressure. The main argument in favour of this may be discerned from the following considerations. The osmotic concentration of the body fluids of animals range from about 0·05 osmole kg^{-1} H_2O in small freshwater animals to about 1 osmole kg^{-1} H_2O in marine invertebrates. A kilogram of water contains about 55·56 moles of water (i.e. 1000 gm/18 gm). Fluid is transported in such a way as to maintain the proportions of water and solute constant in the body fluid. Therefore, in the freshwater animal about 55·51 moles of water must be moved with every 0·05 osmole of solute. Approximately 1100 molecules of water must move with every particle of solute. In the case of marine animals, about 54·6 molecules of water must move with each particle of solute. It may be assumed that it takes as much energy to actively transport a molecule of water as it takes to transport a molecule of solute. Therefore, much less energy need be expended if solute is transported to set up an osmotic gradient down which water will move passively, rather than the reverse.

The kinds of water movement

Movement of water depends upon the energy available to break down its structure. The application of small amounts of energy will cause the hydrogen bonds between water molecules to break down individually and randomly, so that water molecules move individually. Movement will occur in a direction away from the greatest thermal activity (concentration) of the water molecules. This is the familiar process of diffusion. When the energy that is applied is sufficiently large, whole layers (lamina) of structured water will break free from neighboring layers. That is, there will be a bulk breakdown of hydrogen bonds between water molecules so that the layers of water will slide by each other; this is laminar flow. The important difference between diffusion and laminar flow is the linear velocity of the water movement. Flow is very much more rapid than diffusion.

Water movement along the lumena of renal organs is quite clearly a flow process whereby solutes are carried along. However, as has been discussed earlier, water and solutes also move across epithelia and membranes. These offer far greater restriction to movement than does free flow in lumena. Nevertheless, it is now generally considered that here also flow must occur, because of the rapidity of the movement of water. Whilst it seems reasonably certain that flow is involved in transepithelial water (fluid) movement, the energy sources and pathways of this movement are not so clear.

Energy source of fluid movement

Water movement across epithelia in the absence of significant osmotic or hydrostatic pressure gradients appears to be inextricably linked with solute movements; that is, water movement appears to be a passive concomitant of active solute transport. Active solute movement is considered to be mediated by 'carriers' of some kind and cellular energy is expended. The carriers may be large molecules which bind solute on one side of cellular membranes, carry it through the membrane and release it on the other side. Enzymes appear to be involved in some way.

Even though the carrier : solute relationship is poorly understood, the mechanism of active transport of solutes may be treated as a 'black box'. That is, active transport may be described in terms of its effects and the variables that affect it (Chapter 2). It is hoped that what is in the black box will be understood better when more information is available concerning its operating characteristics.

Classically, the black box has been considered to be located in the cell, and solutes and water pass through the cell. Recently, it has been discovered that in many fluid-transporting epithelia extracellular or intracellular spaces exist through which solute and water may move. The investigation of the spaces within or immediately adjacent to cells may reveal little about the actual mechanism of active solute transport. However, they may reveal considerable information about the processes of transepithelial fluid movement. The spaces have been incorporated into recent models of fluid transport, which will be considered below.

Fluid transport across epithelia; theoretical considerations

When fluid moves across epithelia it must penetrate one or both of two kinds of membranes: the plasma membrane of the cell and the basement membrane. The plasma membrane appears to be composed of lipid and protein. In some cases the protein component is composed of glyco-peptide (mucopolysaccharide). Basement membranes appear to be composed entirely of glycopeptide. The passive movement of water and water-soluble solutes through cellular membranes may, therefore, involve pathways in which those substances are insoluble. It is unlikely that water-soluble substances penetrate the lipid portions of the mem-branes. The view is widely held that biological membranes contain water-filled holes or pores through which water and water-soluble substances move.

Even though pores may permit fluid to pass through membranes, they greatly restrict the quantity and quality of that fluid. These restric-tions have been defined for many artificial and some natural membranes. In order to understand the working of the models of fluid transport we will discuss below, it is necessary first briefly to consider the restric-tions to fluid movement offered by porous membranes.

It is well known that the osmotic pressure which can be developed across a semipermiable membrane is proportional to the difference in the number of solute particles on either side of the membrane. By definition, a semipermiable membrane is permeable only to water. Staverman[203] analyzed the effect of porous membranes on the osmotic pressure that could be developed across membranes by solutions containing solute molecules of varying sizes. The osmotic pressure measured across a porous membrane (OP_{meas}) will depart from the theoretical osmotic pressure (OP_{theor}) by a factor which defines the permeability of the membrane to a solute of a particular size. He derived an expression, the 'reflexion coefficient' (σ), which describes the vari-ance from the theoretical of the measured osmotic pressure across a porous membrane (i.e. $\sigma = OP_{meas}/OP_{theor}$). Therefore, if a porous membrane separates two solutions containing solutes to which the membrane is completely impermeable, the measured osmotic pressure will not vary from the theoretical osmotic pressure and sigma (σ) will be unity. If the membrane is completely permeable to solutes, no osmotic pressure will develop and sigma will be equal to zero. Since biological solutions are mixtures of solutes of different sizes the Staverman reflexion coefficients may vary between about one and close to zero.

Of course, the reflexion coefficient is also a statement of the relative velocities of solutes and water through a porous membrane. If the reflexion coefficient is zero, then water and solutes will move through the membrane at equal velocities, If the reflexion coefficient is one, then the velocity of water movement is infinite relative to the velocity of solute movement through a membrane.

A second implication of the porous nature of biological membranes relates to the rate of fluid movement across them. In most animals cells and epithelia water appears to move by flow (called bulk or volume flow) rather than diffusion. The principle support for this view comes from the observation, made repeatedly, that water moves across membranes at a rate well in excess of that expected if diffusive movement alone were involved. The rate of diffusion is independent of pore size where the pore size exceeds the size of the diffusing molecule. However, the rate of flow is critically dependent upon pore size; it is proportional to the square of the radius of the pore.

Pappenheimer[142] has very effectively illustrated the influence of pore size on diffusion and flow as follows. Let us say that two membranes each have a cross-sectional pore area totalling 1 cm². In one membrane there is a single pore of radius, $r = \sqrt{\pi}$ cm. In the other membrane there are 10^4 pores each of a radius, $r = \sqrt{\pi} \times 10^{-2}$ cm. Where the energy gradient is the same, the rate of diffusion through both membranes will be the same. However, where the energy gradient is the same, the rate of flow through the membrane with a single pore will be 10 000 times faster than the rate of flow through the membrane with 10 000 pores.

The water molecule has a radius of about 1·5 Å. When pores approach this dimension, flow will be very restricted; water will move primarily by diffusion. Furthermore, solutes which may accompany the water must themselves approach the size of the water molecule. Most epithelia across which fluid flows behave as if they have pores larger than 1·5 Å. In fact, the calculated pore radii range from about 3 Å to about 50 Å. Pappenheimer[142] has estimated that when pore radii fall below about 20 Å flow will be subjected to greater restriction. Below about 3 Å pore radius, water movement will be primarily of the diffusive type, thus relatively slow.

Models of fluid transport

Four models of fluid transport will be discussed which differ primarily in the nature of the active or energy-requiring step necessary to get water to move passively.

The 'double-membrane' model

The first model of fluid transport which will be considered is that of Curran,[37,38] which is illustrated in Fig. 52a. Curran devised his model to explain movement of fluid from the lumen (mucosa) to the blood (serosa) sides of the small intestine of the rat. He suggested that somewhere in the epithelium there exists a space (2) which is bounded by two membranes (α and β) whose pores have different-sized radii.

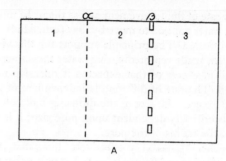

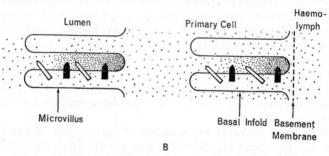

FIG. 52. A. The double-membrane model of fluid transport. Solute is transported into compartment 2, establishing an osmotic gradient across membrane α because the reflexion coefficent of the solute for that membrane is > o; no osmotic gradient exists between compartments 2 and 3 because the reflexion coefficient of the solute for membrane β is zero. Water enters compartment 2 from compartment 1, establishing an hydrostatic pressure which forces fluid into compartment 3. B. The standing-gradient osmotic flow model applied to the Malpighian tubules of *Calliphora*: potassium is actively transported out of basal channels into the adjacent cytoplasm, diluting the fluid toward the closed ends of the channels. Water then flows out of the closed ends of the channels into the adjacent cytoplasm. At the apical border potassium is actively transported out of the cytoplasm in the microvilli into the adjacent lumenal space between the microvilli. This dilutes the cytoplasm toward the closed ends of the microvilli and water flows into the lumenal space making it isosmotic. A. from Curran.[37] B. from Berridge and Oschman.[21]

The pores of membrane α are sufficiently small so that an osmotic pressure gradient will develop across that membrane (i.e. σ is greater than zero for small solutes such as sodium). The pores of β are sufficiently large so that no osmotic pressure will develop across the membrane (i.e. $\sigma = o$ for small solutes). He envisaged that solute is actively transported into compartment 2 from compartment 1. The reflexion coefficient of membrane α for the solute is greater than zero, whilst the reflexion coefficient of membrane β is zero. Therefore, no osmotic pressure difference will exist across membrane β but an osmotic pressure will exist across membrane α. Water will be attracted into space 2 from space 1. If space 2 is not expansible, a hydrostatic pressure will build up there as water enters from space 1. The hydrostatic pressure will force fluid through membrane β whose larger pores offer less restriction to flow. Therefore, there will be a net transfer of fluid from space 1 to space 3.

In the small intestine (ileum) of the rat it appears that sodium is actively transported into the *in vivo* equivalent of space 2 (whatever that may be) and water follows passively. Curran and McIntosh[39] have shown that the model illustrated in Fig. 52a will function if sucrose is placed in space 2. A dialysis membrane which had a σ of 0·1 for sucrose was substituted for membrane α and a sintered glass disc was substituted for membrane β. Under these conditions fluid moved from space 1 to space 3 whenever the osmotic concentration of space 2 exceeded that of space 1.

Curran's model has been applied by other investigators to their preparations. Sodium may be actively transported into intercellular spaces at the lateral borders of the urinary bladder of the toad. Similarly, potassium may be transported into intercellular spaces in the rectum of the blowfly (Fig. 29a) p. 98. In both cases, water will move passively down an osmotic gradient established by active ion transport.[15]

Standing gradient osmotic flow

Diamond and his co-workers, Tormey and Bossert,[43–45,212] have developed a model based on a functional geometry within fluid-transporting epithelia. It depends upon channels which are structurally or functionally closed at one end. The channels are found within or adjacent to fluid-transporting cells. Solute is pumped into the closed ends of the spaces from the adjacent cytoplasm, making the region hyperosmotic to the cell. Water moves into the space from the adjacent cytoplasm so that toward the open end of the space, the fluid is isosmotic to the cytoplasm. In effect, a standing osmotic gradient is established along the length of the channel at equilibrium. Fluid will move out of the open end of the channel. By varying the geometry of the channel, the fluid which moves out of the open end may vary in its osmotic concentration. If the channel is short and wide there will be less time for osmotic equilibrium between the cytoplasm and channel to be established. Thus the fluid that will flow out of the open end will be hyperosmotic to the cytoplasm. If the channel is long and narrow, osmotic equilibrium between channel and cytoplasm will be established and the fluid which flows out of the open end will be isosmotic to the cytoplasm. The channels may be found at the bases of the cells, the lateral membranes or even between the apical microvilli.

Diamond's model has been derived from studies of the rabbit gallbladder. It has been applied by Diamond and others to other fluid-transporting epithelia. Recently, Berridge and Oschman[21] have utilized the model to explain fluid 'secretion' by the Malpighian tubules of the blowfly, *Calliphora*. Electron micrographs of the blowfly Malpighian tubules reveal extensive basal channels (Fig. 19 p. 77). Berridge and Oschman suggested that potassium is actively transported out of these spaces, diluting the fluid toward their closed ends (Fig. 52b). Water may then move passively into the adjacent cytoplasm, which is made hypertonic by transport of potassium out of the spaces. At the apical region of the cell, potassium is transported out of the cytoplasm of the microvilli into the lumenal space between the microvilli, concentrating that space. Water then moves passively out of the cytoplasm so that toward the open end of the spaces between the microvilli, the fluid is again isosmotic.

Wall and Oschman[223] have suggested that the standing gradient model may explain fluid transport by the rectal pads of the cockroach, *Periplaneta* (Chapter 8). Active transport of solute (sodium) into intercellular channels may attract water out of the cells leading to a flow of fluid into intercellular spaces and out of the rectal pad epithelium. Water is attracted out of the rectal lumen by the hyperosmoticity of the cells resulting from loss of water to the intercellular channels. (See Chapter 8 for a fuller discussion).

'Volume pump' model

It can be seen that the double membrane and standing gradient osmotic flow models are very similar. Both require two barriers to solute movement which are placed in series. However, they differ primarily in the permeability of the first barrier. A third model was recently devised by Frederiksen and Leyssac,[53] and is also based on studies of the isolated rabbit gall bladder. Frederiksen and Leyssac found that under certain conditions there appeared to be no direct relationship between the rate of fluid transport by the gall bladder and the rate of sodium transport. This seemed to suggest that sodium transport was not always directly linked to fluid movement, an essential feature of both the 'double membrane' and 'standing gradient' models. Again, at variance with other studies, Frederiksen and Leyssac found that the rate of oxygen consumption of the gall bladder varied in direct proportion to the rate of fluid transport, and inversely with the rate of sodium transport. These studies seemed to indicate that the main energy-requiring step in fluid transport by the gall-bladder is related to the mechanism of moving the fluid, but this mechanism is not necessarily active solute (Na) transport.

In order to explain their results, they constructed a model which could be compatible both with their results and with certain ultra-structural features of many fluid-transporting epithelia. They hypothesized that fluid movement is underlain by a 'mechanical volume pump' (Fig. 53), which 'pumps' fluid from the apical region of the cell to the lateral border of the cells, where it is released into the intercellular space. They suggested that the systems of microtubules and microvesicles seen in electron micrographs of fluid-transporting cells may be involved.

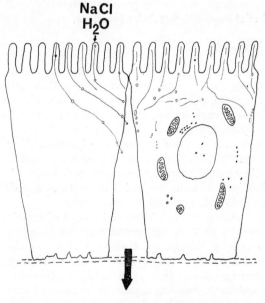

Fig. 53. The volume-pump model. Solute and water are taken up from the lumen at the apical membrane as a 'unit volume' and mechanically propulsed through the apical cytoplasm of the cell. Unit volumes move within a structural network of fine tubules and/or vesicles. The fluid is released into the intercellular space where hydrostatic pressure causes it to move across the basement membrane (dashed line). From Frederiksen and Leyssac.[53]

The actual operation of the volume-pump model is entirely a matter for speculation. Frederiksen and Leyssac suggested that the initial step in transcellular fluid transport is an interaction between the apical cell membrance and the transported solute (e.g. Na^+, Cl^-, other monovalent anions). In some way this induces a localized 'weakness' in the apical cell membrane which may take the form of an invagination or perhaps a pore. In any event, the interaction results in the uptake of a certain amount of fluid which is isosmotic with, but not necessarily identical in composition to, the fluid bathing the apical membrane of the cell. The fluid is isolated in an intracellular compartment as a 'unit volume' initially; the unit volume is mechanically propulsed through the apical cytoplasm within the substructural system (e.g. microtubules) to the lateral border, where it is released into the intercellular space. This creates an hydrostatic pressure in the relatively restricted intercellular space and the fluid flows across the basement membrane due to the pressure differential and the 'impermeability' of the apical intercellular junctions.

'Formed-body' model

As outlined in Chapter 9, the antennal gland of the crayfish and other organs produce small formed elements within their cells which are extruded from the cells to lie free in the extracellular space. These formed elements vary considerably in size and morphology so they have been given the general apellation, 'formed bodies'. There is evidence that at least some of them are lysosomes.[175,180] *In vitro* studies of the behaviour of formed bodies reveal that they may be implicated in transepithelial fluid movements (Chapter 9). Therefore, a model has been constructed which attempts to explain the rôle of formed bodies in transepithelial fluid movement.

Formed bodies probably arise by vesiculation of the cell membrane; the small vesicles thus formed may or may not be incorporated into larger intracellular structures. Formed bodies contain hydrolytic enzymes, and it is known that hydrolysis occurs within them.[175] The formed bodies are released into spaces within or adjacent to cells where they swell and burst. Swelling appears to be caused by the movement of water into them, probably due to the osmotic attraction of products of hydrolysis. However, the water which moves into the swelling formed bodies does not appear to be accompanied by solutes. Therefore, solutes tend to become concentrated in the medium surrounding them.[179] When the formed bodies have swollen to a critical size they burst.[175,176,177-180A]

The mechanism of fluid flow caused by the swelling of formed bodies is depicted schematically in Fig. 54a. Formed bodies are extruded from the cytoplasm of the cells into a space (C) where free water is available. They take up water and swell, concentrating solute in space C. This sets up a movement of fluid into space C from spaces A and B. Space C is relatively indistensible so that the movement of fluid into it creates an hydrostatic pressure within. Fluid moves out of space C in a direction determined by the restriction to flow of passages α and β. In the diagram passage β is less restricted than is passage α so that fluid will flow from space A to space B.

The formed-body model differs from the double-membrane and standing-osmotic-gradient models primarily in the mechanism used

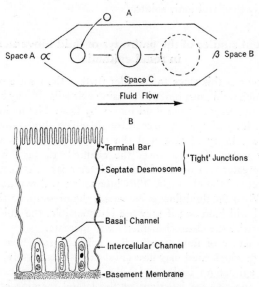

FIG. 54. A. The formed-body model of fluid transport. Formed bodies are extruded from the cytoplasm of cells into spaces where they swell, taking up water, and concentrating the medium surrounding them. Water enters the formed-body space (C) from adjacent spaces A and B, creating an hydrostatic pressure which forces fluid out of space C in a direction determined by the resistance to flow of passages α and β. In the diagram, passage β is less restricted than is passage α, so that fluid will flow from space A to space B. The formed bodies burst after they have swollen to a critical size. B. Possible formed-body swelling spaces and passages offering resistance to fluid flow in a 'typical' epithelial cell. From Riegel.[180]

to localize solute. In order that solutes be localized in intracellular or extracellular spaces, access to those spaces must be restricted. The restriction must be sufficiently great that solutes will not rapidly diffuse or flow away. If the solutes providing the osmotic driving force are small, ions of the size of, say, sodium (hydrated radius $\simeq 2 \cdot 56 \, \text{Å}$[201]), the access passages will have to be quite small. This will restrict the rate at which fluid will flow. If the solute providing the osmotic driving force is enclosed in a formed body which is of microscopic dimensions, the access passages need be only small enough to retain the formed bodies in the swelling space until they have burst. Extracellularly, formed bodies may be several microns in diameter. Therefore formed bodies swelling in enclosed spaces will permit fluid to flow very much more rapidly than will ionic solutes.

Recent studies of the pathways of fluid movement in renal epithelia

It is pertinent at this stage to consider further the nature of passages through which fluid must move in crossing epithelia. It may be assumed that in the majority of cases fluid moves by flow. The main effects of the size (radius) of the passages through which fluid moves will be seen in the velocity of flow and the size of the solutes which will accompany water. The narrower the channels through which fluid flows, the greater will be the frictional interactions between the fluid and the walls of the channels. This interaction will manifest itself as pressure. When the fluid flow is increased, the pressure on the walls of the channel will increase; if they are indistensible, the fluid will flow faster, otherwise the channel diameter will increase.

The structure of fluid-transporting epithelia reveals at least four sites through which fluid may flow (Fig. 54b). These are (1) the lumen which the epithelium encloses, (2) the basement membrane, (3) the cell membrane and (4) junctions at the lateral margins of the cells. Lumena in renal organs range from a few microns to several millimetres or centimetres. Therefore, they will offer no restriction to the passage of dissolved solutes, but they may restrict the flow of fluid. The basement membrane restricts both fluid flow and the passage of solutes; its effects may be seen principally, however, in the restriction it offers to solute movement. In general, the basement membranes of various cells seem to allow relatively free passage of molecules whose radii are of the order of 20 Å or less. Cell membranes place a very severe restriction on both fluid flow and solute movement. They behave as if they have pores of a radius of only a few Ångstroms (e.g. $3 \cdot 5$ to $4 \cdot 2 \, \text{Å}$[201]). It has been considered that the junctional complexes between cells are impermeable to fluid. In electron micrographs it is possible to see that the lateral membranes of cells are very close together, especially at apical 'tight' junctions. The spaces between the membranes may be no more than ten Ångstroms or the outer members of the cell membranes may be 'fused'. However, the existence of fluid-tight barriers between some cells may be thrown into doubt by recent studies. For example, the 'apparent reflexion coefficients' of water-soluble non-electrolytes in proximal tubules of *Necturus* were estimated using the stopped-flow microperfusion technique.[8] Despite wide variation in the size of molecules in solutions perfused into the tubules, the apparent reflexion coefficients were remarkably similar (Table 25). From these results it was concluded

TABLE 25

Apparent reflexion coefficients of water-soluble non-electrolytes in the proximal tubule of Necturus. *Slightly modified from Bentzel, Davis, Scott, Zatzman and Solomon.*[8]

	Substance	Molecular weight	Molecular radius (Å)*	Apparent reflection coeff.**
GROUP 1	Glycerol	92	2·78	0·38
	Diethylene Glycol	106	2·73	0·47
	Erythritol	122	2·89	0·50
	Mannitol	182	3·15	0·79
	Tetraethylene Glycol	194	3·78	0·51
	Raffinose	594	4·62	0·51
GROUP 2	Polyethylene Glycol	400	6·1	0·56
	,, ,,	1000	9·7	0·56
	,, ,,	4000	19·4	0·52
	,, ,,	6000	23·7	0·71

* Method of determining the molecular radii of substances in the two groups was different, therefore the radii are not strictly comparable, except within the group.
** The standard error of these determinations was estimated to be ±10%.[8]

that the barrier to solute movement across the proximal tubule epithelium of *Necturus* cannot distinguish between molecules solely on the basis of size (molecular radius). Therefore, the barrier must be more complex than, say, a simple pore. Furthermore, apertures sufficiently large to permit molecules listed in Table 25 to pass would not permit the cells to maintain their integrity. From this evidence it was concluded that the route of fluid flow was between the cells.[8] Since the cells in the proximal tubule of *Necturus* are joined by apical junctional complexes, the possibility exists that such 'tight junctions' are not so 'tight' as was believed originally.

Another possible route of fluid movement through intercellular spaces arises from the studies of Bulger and Trump.[77] Indian ink (colloidal carbon) injected into the lumen of the nephrons of the English sole appears in the intercellular spaces. This seemed to be the result of uptake of fluid from the nephron lumen by 'massive invaginations' of the lumenal membranes, which then fuse with the lateral membrane basal to the apical tight junctions between the cells. Therefore, the route of fluid movement 'bypasses' the tight junctions.

Extracellular spaces have been seen in electron micrographs of collecting ducts and proximal and distal tubules of mammals. In the isolated, perfused collecting ducts of rabbits, the width of the spaces varies according to whether or not anti-diuretic hormone (ADH) is present in the medium bathing the tubules. When ADH is present, the spaces become enlarged and the cells appear to swell[57]. As discussed in Chapter 6, ADH increases the permeability of collecting ducts, and it is probable that this is due to increased extracellular fluid movement. the iron-containing protein, ferritin, can be forced to enter the basal and lateral extracellular spaces in the proximal and distal tubules of the rat nephron if the pressure in the peritubular capillaries is elevated. The ferritin molecule has a radius of about 55 Å; this indicates that the basement membrane of the tubule cells is permeable, at least under pressure, to quite large molecules. The ferritin did not appear in the lumen of the tubules, so perhaps the apical junctional complexes are not permeable to molecules of such a size. Probably the most interesting finding of this study, at least in the context of the present chapter, is that the intercellular spaces have the same density as the cytoplasm. This suggested that organic material may be present in the intercellular spaces.[207]

Electrical studies have also provided evidence for an extracellular pathway of fluid movement in the proximal tubules of amphibians. Boulpaep,[28] and Hoshi and Sakai[80] have demonstrated that there is an extracellular electrical shunt pathway which significantly lowers the transtubular electrical potential difference. This may also be deduced from the observations that the perfusion of tubule lumena with non-penetrating electrolytes causes a large increase in the transtubular potential (e.g. Fig. 11, p. 42, distal tubule with sulphate added).

Schmidt-Nielsen and Davis[187] have summarized studies of fluid movement and intercellular channels in reptile kidneys. They studied the ultrastructural appearance of the intercellular channels in the proximal and distal tubules under normal conditions and during diuresis and anti-diuresis. In normal animals the spaces at the lateral margins of the cells of the proximal tubules may be closed or they may exhibit varying degrees of patency. Spaces at the lateral margins of cells of the distal tubule are generally open under normal conditions. When the animals are experimentally made diuretic or anti-diuretic, only two consistent relationships could be seen which related to the degree of patency of the intercellular spaces. First, when fluid movement was halted because the lumen of the tubule was collapsed or because transepithelial fluid movement was, presumably, poisoned with ouabain, the spaces were wholly or partially closed. Secondly, in dehydrated animals, the spaces in the distal tubule were abnormally large. Under conditions of dehydration it would be expected that maximum fluid reabsorption across the epithelium of the distal tubule would be occurring.

Studies have been made of the effects of hydration and dehydration on extracellular spaces in the recta of insects. In the blowfly, *Calliphora*, the intercellular spaces between the cortical cells of the rectal papillae are very extensive (Fig. 29a, p. 98). In blowflies that are feeding normally, the intercellular spaces were highly dilated. Reabsorption of potassium and water from the rectum in such flies was very rapid, suggesting that the spaces were dilated due to active water and ion reabsorption. Injection of a solution which was hypoosmotic to the haemolymph caused dilation of the intercellular spaces. In fasting flies or starved flies, the intercellular spaces of the cortical cells were collapsed. Presumably the rectal papillae are relatively inactive in starved or fasting flies. It was therefore assumed that the collapsed spaces indicate that little fluid reabsorption was occurring.[19] Berridge and Gupta suggested that solute-linked water movement in the rectal papillae of *Calliphora* conforms to Curran's model. They suggested that membranous stacks at the lateral plasma membranes 'pump' ions into the intercellular spaces and that water follows passively. Berridge and Gupta found also that after injection of distilled water into the rectum, an electron-dense material, probably organic in nature, appeared in the intercellular spaces.

Grimstone, Mullinger and Ramsay[69] have noted extensive 'extracellular' spaces at the bases of the cells of those parts of the Malpighian tubule which participate in the rectal complex of *Tenebrio*. (Chapter 8). The spaces could be closed or open, but there seemed to be so much variation between cells of individual tubules taken from hydrated and dehydrated animals that the investigators were loath to speculate as to their significance.

It is clear that extracellular pathways of transepithelial fluid movement exist, but the exact nature and extent of these pathways are yet to be fully explored. Electron micrographs must be interpreted with caution because channels and spaces may widen or narrow by the simple act of varying the osmotic concentration of the solutions used to fix the tissues. Nevertheless, spaces have been observed to vary in width in living tissue (e.g. rabbit gall bladder[45]). Therefore, it is likely that not all instances of spaces seen in electron micrographs are artifactual.

The few examples that we have cited here may serve to illustrate that renal physiology may be moving out of the 'black box' stage, at least with respect to the cell and its environment. The next few years may well see a considerable advance in our understanding of the functional significance of ultrastructure. During this advance it would be surprising if some of our most cherished ideas are not subjected to close critical scrutiny and found to be inadequate.

References

1. ANDERSON, E., and BEAMS, H. W. 1956. Light and electron microscope studies on the cells of the labyrinth in the green gland of *Cambarus* sp. *Proc. Iowa Acad. Sci.*, **64**, 681–685.
2. BAHL, K. N. 1947. Excretion in the oligochaeta. *Biol. Rev.*, **22**, 109–147.
3. BEAMS, H. W., ANDERSON, E., and PRESS, N. 1956. Light and electron microscope studies on the cells of the distal portion of the crayfish nephron tubule. *Cytologia*, **21**, 50–57.
4. — TAHMISIAN, T. N., and DEVINE, R. L. 1955. Electron microscope studies on the cells of the Malpighian tubules of the grasshopper (Orthoptera, Acrididae). *J. Biophys. Biochem. Cytol.*, **1**, 197–202.
5. BENNETT, C. M., CLAPP, J. R., and BERLINER, R. W. 1967. Micropuncture study of the proximal and distal tubule in the dog. *Am. J. Physiol.*, **213**, 1254–1262.
6. — BRENNER, B. M., and BERLINER, R. W. 1968. Micropuncture study of nephron function in the Rhesus monkey. *J. clin. Invest.*, **47**, 203–216.
7. BENTLEY, P. J. 1966. The physiology of the urinary bladder of amphibia. *Biol. Rev.*, **41**, 275–316.
8. BENTZEL, C. J., DAVIS, M., *et al.* 1968. Osmotic volume flow in the proximal tubule of *Necturus* kidney. *J. gen. Physiol.*, **51**, 517–533.
9. BERLINER, R. W. 1959/1960. Renal mechanisms for potassium excretion. *Harvey Lectures*, **55**, 141–171.
10. — KENNEDY, T. J., and ORLOFF, J. 1951. Relationship between acidification of the urine and potassium metabolism. Effect of carbonic anhydrase inhibition on potassium excretion. *Am. J. Med.*, **11**, 274–282.
11. — LEVINSKY, N. G., *et al.* 1958. Dilution and concentration of the urine and action of anti-diuretic hormone. *Am. J. Med.*, **24**, 730–744.
12. BERRIDGE, M. J. 1965. The physiology of excretion in the cotton stainer, *Dysdercus fasciatus* Signoret. I–III. *J. exp. Biol.*, **43**, 511–552.
13. — 1966a. The physiology of excretion in the cotton stainer, *Dysdercus fasciatus* Signoret. IV. Hormonal control of excretion. *J. exp. Biol.*, **44**, 553–566.
14. — 1966b. Metabolic pathways of isolated Malpighian tubules of the blowfly functioning in an artificial medium. *J. Insect Physiol.*, **12**, 1523–1538.
15. — 1967. Ion and water transport across epithelia. In *Insects and physiology*. J. W. L. Beament, and J. E. Treherne (Eds). Oliver and Boyd, Edinburgh.
16. — 1968. Urine formation by the Malpighian tubules of *Calliphora*. I. Cations. *J. exp. Biol.*, **48**, 159–174.

17. BERRIDGE, M. J. 1969. Urine formation by the Malpighian tubules of *Calliphora*. II. Anions. *J. exp. Biol.*, **50**, 15–28.

18. — 1970. Osmoregulation in terrestrial arthropods. In *Chemical zoology*, **5**, M. Florkin and B. T. Scheer (Eds). Academic Press, London and New York.

19. — and GUPTA, B. L. 1967. Fine-structural changes in relation to ion and water transport in the rectal papillae of the blowfly, *Calliphora*. *J. Cell Sci.*, **2**, 89–112.

21. — and OSCHMAN, J. L. 1969. A structural basis for fluid secretion by Malpighian tubules. *Tissue and Cell*, **1**, 247–272.

22. BINNS, R. 1969. The physiology of the antennal gland of *Carcinus maenas* (L.). I–V. *J. exp. Biol.*, **51**, 1–45.

23. BOROFFKA, I. 1965. Elektrolyttransport im Nephridium von *Lumbricus terrestris*. *Z. vergl. Physiol.*, **51**, 25–48.

24. — ALTNER, H., and HAUPT, J. 1970. Funktion und Ultrastruktur des Nephridiums von *Hirudo medicinalis*. I. Ort und Mechanismus der Primärharnbildung. *Z. vergl. Physiol.*, **66**, 421–438.

25. BORRADAILE, L. A., EASTHAM, L. E. S., *et al.* 1961. *The Invertebrata*, 4th edn, rev. by G. A. Kerkut. Cambridge Univ. Press.

26. BOTT, P. A. 1962. Micropuncture study of renal excretion of water, K, Na, and Cl in *Necturus*. *Am. J. Physiol.*, **203**, 662–666.

28. BOULPAEP, E. L. 1967. Ion permeability of the peritubular and lumenal membrane of the renal tubular cell. In *Transport und Funktion Intracellulärer Elektrolyte*. Urban and Schwarzenberg, Berlin.

29. BRAUN, G., KÜMMEL, G., and MANGOS, J. A. 1966. Studies on the ultrastructure and function of a primitive excretory organ, the protonephridium of the rotifer, *Asplanchna priodonta*. *Pflüg. Arch.*, **289**, 141–154.

30. BRYAN, G. W. 1965. Ionic regulation in the squat lobster *Galathea squamifera*, with special reference to the relationship between potassium metabolism and the accumulation of radioactive caesium. *J. mar. biol. Ass. U.K.*, **45**, 97–102.

31. — and WARD, E. 1962. Potassium metabolism and the accumulation of Caesium[137] by decapod Crustacea. *J. mar. biol. Ass. U.K.*, **42**, 199–241.

32. BURGER, J. W. 1957. The general form of excretion in the lobster, *Homarus*. *Biol. Bull. Woods Hole*, **113**, 207–223.

32A. CAPELLI, J. P., WESSON, L. G. Jnr., and APONTE, G. E. 1970. A phylogenic study of the renin-angiotensin system. *Am. J. Physiol.*, **218**, 1171–1178.

33. CARONE, F. A., EVERETT, B. A., *et al.* 1967. Renal localization of albumen and its function in the concentrating mechanism. *Am. J. Physiol.*, **212**, 387–393.

34. CARTER, G. S. 1951. *General zoology of the invertebrates*. Sidgwick and Jackson, London.

35. CHINARD, F. P. 1964. Kidney, water and electrolytes. *A. Rev. Physiol.*, **26**, 187–226.

36. — VOSBURGH, G. J., and ENNS, T. 1955. Transcapillary exchange of water and of other substances in certain organs of the dog. *Am. J. Physiol.*, **183**, 221–234.

37. CURRAN, P. F. 1960. Na, Cl, and water transport by rat ileum *in vitro. J. gen Physiol.*, **43**, 1137–1148.

38. — 1965. Ion transport in intestine and its coupling to other transport processes. *Fedn Proc. Fedn Am. Socs exp. Biol.*, **24**, 993–999.

39. — and MCINTOSH, J. R. 1962. *Nature, Lond.*, **193**, 347.

40. DANIELLI, J. F., and PANTIN, C. F. A. 1960. Alkaline phosphatase in protonephridia of terrestrial nemertines and planarians. *Q. Jl. microsc. Sci.*, **91**, 209–213.

41. DAVSON, H. 1964. *Textbook of general physiology*. Churchill, London.

42. — and DANIELLI, J. F. 1952. *The permeability of natural membranes*. Cambridge Univ. Press.

43. DIAMOND, J. M., and BOSSERT, W. H. 1967. Standing-gradient osmotic flow. A mechanism for coupling of water and solute transport in epithelia. *J. gen. Physiol.*, **50**, 2061–2083.

44. — and — 1968. Functional consequences of ultrastructural geometry in 'backwards' fluid-transporting epithelia. *J. Cell Biol.*, **37**, 694–702.

45. — and TORMEY, J. McD. 1966. Role of long extracellular channels in fluid transport across epithelia. *Nature, Lond.*, **210**, 817–820.

46. — and WRIGHT, E. M. 1969. Biological membranes: The physical basis of ion and nonelectrolyte selectivity. *A. Rev. Physiol.*, **31**, 581–646.

46A. DICKER, S. E. 1970. Mechanisms of urine concentration and dilution in mammals. Monograph of the *Physiological Society No. 20*. Edward Arnold, London.

47. EIGLER, F. W. 1961. Short-circuit current measurements in proximal tubule of *Necturus* kidney. *Am. J. Physiol.*, **201**, 157–163.

48. FEUSTEL, H. 1958. Untersuchungen uber die Exkretion bei Collembolen. *Z. wiss. Zool.*, **161**, 209–238.

49. FLORKIN, M. 1938. Contribution a l'etude de l'osmoregulation chez les Invertebres d'eau douce. I. *Arch. Internat. Physiol.*, **47**, 113–124.

50. — and DUCHATEAU, G. 1948. Sur l'osmoregulation de l'Anodonte (*Anodonta cygnea* L.). *Physiol. Comp. Oecol.*, **1**, 29–45.

51. FORSTER, R. F. 1961. Kidney Cells. In *The cell*. J. Brachet and A. E. Mirsky (Eds). Academic Press, New York.

52. FORSTER, R. P., and HONG, S. K. 1962. Tubular transport maxima of *PAH* and Diodrast measured individually in the aglomerular kidney of *Lophius*, and simultaneously as competitors under conditions of equimolar loading. *J. gen. Physiol.*, **45**, 811–820.

53. FREDERIKSEN, O., and LEYSSAC, P. P. 1969. Transcellular transport of isosmotic volumes by the rabbit gall-bladder *in vitro. J. Physiol.*, **201,** 201–224.

54. FRETTER, V., and GRAHAM, A. 1962. *British prosobranch molluscs.* Ray Society, London.

55. FRÖMTER, W., and HEGEL, U. 1966. Transtubuläre Potentialdifferenzen an proximalen und distalen Tubuli der Rattenniere. *Arch. ges. Physiol.*, **291,** 107–120.

56. FÜLGRAFF, G., and HEIDENREICH, O. 1967. Mikropunktionsuntersuchungen über die Wirkung von Calciumionen auf die Resorptionskapazität und auf die prozentuale Resorption im proximalen Konvolut von Ratten. *Arch. Exp. Pharmakol. Pathol.*, **258,** 440–451.

57. GANOTE, C. E., GRANTHAM, J. J., *et al.* 1968. Ultrastructural studies of vasopressin effect on isolated perfused renal collecting tubules of the rabbit. *J. Cell Biol.*, **36,** 355–367.

58. GIEBISCH, G. 1958. Electrical potential measurements on single nephrons of Necturus. *J. Cell. Comp. Physiol*, **51,** 221–239.

59. — WINDHAGER, E. E., and PITTS, R. F. 1960. Mechanism of urinary acidification. In: *Biology of Pyelonephritis.* Quinn, E. L. and Kass, E. M. (Eds). Churchill, London.

60. — and — 1964. Renal tubular transfer of sodium, chloride and potassium. *Am. J. Med.*, **36,** 643–669.

61. — KLOSE, R. M., *et al.* 1964. Sodium movement across single perfused proximal tubules of rat kidneys. *J. gen. Physiol.*, **47,** 1175–1194.

62. GOODRICH, E. S. 1945. The study of nephridia and genital ducts since 1895. *Q. Jl. microsc. Sci.*, **88,** 113–301.

63. — 1958. *Studies on the structure and development of vertebrates,* **2,** Chap. 13. Constable, London.

64. GOTTSCHALK, C. W. 1962/1963. Renal tubular function: lessons from micropuncture. *Harvey Lectures*, **58,** 95–124.

65. — 1964. Osmotic concentration and dilution of the urine. *Am. J. Med.*, **36,** 670–685.

66. — LASSITER, W. W., and MYLLE, M. 1960. Localization of urine acidification in the mammalian kidney. *Am. J. Physiol.*, **198,** 581–585.

67. — and MYLLE, M. 1959. Micropuncture study of the mammalian urinary concentrating mechanism. *Am. J. Physiol.*, **196,** 927–936.

68. GRASZYNSKI, K. 1963. Die Feinstrukur des Nephridialkanals von *Lumbricus terrestris* L. Eine elektronen mikroskopische Untersuchung. *Zool. Beitr.* (N. F.) **8,** 189–296.

69. GRIMSTONE, A. V., MULLINGER, A. M., and RAMSAY, J. A. 1968. Further studies on the rectal complex of the mealworm, *Tenebrio molitor* L. (Coleoptera, Tenebrionidae). *Phil. Trans. R. Soc., Lond.*, B, **253,** 343–382.

70. GROSS, W. J. 1967. Glucose absorption from the urinary bladder of a crab. *Comp. Biochem. Physiol.*, **20,** 313–317.

71. GUPTA, B. L., and BERRIDGE, M. J. 1966. Fine structural organization of the rectum of the blowfly, *Calliphora erythrocephala* (Meig.) with special reference to connective tissue, tracheae and neurosecretory innervation in the rectal papillae. *J. Morph.*, **120**, 23–82.

72. HAECKEL, R., HESS, B., et al. 1968. Purification and allosteric properties of yeast pyruvate kinase. *Hoppe-Seyler's Z. physiol. Chem.*, **349**, 699–714.

73. HARDWICKE, J., HULME, B., et al. 1968. The measurement of glomerular permeability to polydisperse radioactively-labelled macromolecules in normal rabbits. *Clin. Sci.*, **34**, 505–514.

74. HARRISON, F. M. 1962. Some excretory processes in the abalone, *Haliotis rufescens. J. exp. Biol.*, **39**, 179–182.

75. — and MARTIN, A. W. 1965. Excretion in the cephalopod, *Octopus dolfleini. J. exp. Biol.*, **42**, 71–98.

76. HAYMAN, J. Quoted in ref. 41.

77. HICKMAN, C. P., Jnr., and TRUMP, B. F. 1969. The Kidney, In *Fish physiology*, **1**, Hoar, W., and Randall, P. (Eds). Academic Press, London and New York.

78. HILGER, H. H., KLÜMPER, J. D., and ULLRICH, K. J. 1958. Wasserrückresorption und Ionentransport durch die Sammelrohrzellen der Säugetierniere. *Pflüg. Arch.*, **267**, 218–237.

79. HORSTER, M., and THURAU, K. 1968. Micropuncture studies on the filtration rate of single superficial and juxtamedullary glomeruli in the rat kidney. *Pflüg. Arch.*, **301**, 162–181.

80. HOSHI, T., and SAKAI, F. 1967. A comparison of the electrical resistance of the surface cell membrane and cellular wall in the proximal tubule of the newt kidney. *Japan. J. Physiol.*, **17**, 627–637.

81. HOUSSAY, B. A., LEWIS, J. T., et al. 1951. *Human physiology*. McGraw-Hill, London and New York.

82. HUANG, R., HUTTON, L., and KALANT, N. 1967. Molecular sieving by glomerular basement membrane. *Nature, Lond.*, **216**, 87–88.

83. IRVINE, H. B. 1969. Sodium and potassium secretion by isolated insect Malpighian tubules. *Am. J. Physiol.*, **217**, 1520–1527.

84. JAENIKE, J. R., and BERLINER, R. W. 1960. A study of distal renal tubular functions by a modified stop flow technique. *J. clin. Invest.*, **39**, 481–490.

85. JAMISON, R. L. 1968. Micropuncture study of segments of thin loop of Henle in the rat. *Am. J. Physiol.*, **215**, 236–242.

86. — BENNETT, C. M., and BERLINER, R. W. 1967. Countercurrent multiplication by the thin loops of Henle. *Am. J. Physiol.*, **212**, 357–366.

87. KAMEMOTO, F. I., KEISTER, S. M., and SPALDING, A. E. 1962. Cholinesterase activities and sodium movement in the crayfish kidney. *Comp. Biochem. Physiol.*, **7**, 81–87.

88. KAMEMOTO, F. I., SPALDING, A. E., and KEISTER, S. M. 1962. Ionic balance in blood and coelomic fluid of earthworms. *Biol. Bull. Woods Hole*, **122**, 228–231.

88A. KEEFE, P. A. Personal communication.

89. KIRSCHNER, L. B. 1967. Invertebrate excretory organs. *A. Rev. Physiol.*, **29**, 169–196.

90. — and WAGNER, S. 1965. The site and permeability of the filtration locus in the crayfish antennal gland. *J. exp. Biol.*, **43**, 385–395.

91. KITCHING, J. A. 1967. Contractile vacuoles, ionic regulation and excretion. In *Research in protozoology*, **1**. Pergamon Press, Oxford.

92. KRIZ, W. 1967. Der Architektonische und funktionelle Aufbau der Rattenniere. *Z. Zellforsch.* (*Histochemie*), **82**, 495–535.

93. KÜMMEL, G. 1964. Das Cölomsäckchen der Antennendrüse von *Cambarus affinis* Say (Decapoda, Crustacea). *Zool. Beitr.*, **10**, 227–252.

94. — 1965. Druckfiltration als ein Mechanismus der Stoffausscheidung bei Wirbellosen. In: *Sekretion und Exkretion*. 2. Wiss. Konferenz. d. Ges. Deut. Naturforscher u. Arzte, Schloss Reinhardsbrunn b. Friedrichroda 1964. Springer-Verlag, Berlin.

95. LATTA, H., MAUNSBACH, A. B., and OSVALDO, L. 1967. The fine structure of renal tubules in cortex and medulla. In *Ultrastructure of the kidney*. Academic Press, London and New York.

96. LAVERACK, M. S. 1963. *The physiology of earthworms*. Pergamon Press, Oxford.

97. LEAF, A. 1960. Some actions of neurohypophyseal hormones on a living membrane. *J. gen. Physiol.*, **43**, (Suppl.) 175–189.

98. LE BRIE, S. J. 1968. Renal lymph and osmotic diuresis. *Am. J. Physiol.*, **215**, 116–123.

99. — and MAYERSON, H. S. 1960. Influence of elevated venous pressure on flow and composition of renal lymph. *Am. J. Physiol.*, **198**, 1037–1040.

100. LEWY, J., and WINDHAGER, E. E. 1968. Peritubular control of proximal tubular fluid reabsorption in the rat kidney. *Am. J. Physiol.*, **214**, 943–954.

100A. LEYSSAC, P. P. 1966. The regulation of proximal tubular reabsorption in the mammalian kidney. *Acta Physiol. Scand.*, **70**, (suppl. 291), 1–151.

101. LISON, L. 1942. Recherches sur l'histophysiology comparée de l'excretion chez les Arthropodes. *Mem. Acad. Belg.*, *Ser. 2 cl. Sci.*, **19**, 1–107.

102. LITCHFIELD, J. B., and BOTT, P. A. 1962. Micropuncture study of renal excretion of water, K, Na, and Cl in the rat. *Am. J. Physiol.*, **203**, 667–670.

103. LITTLE, C. 1965. The formation of urine by the prosobranch gastropod mollusc *Viviparus viviparus* Linn. *J. exp. Biol.*, **43**, 39–54.

104. LOCKWOOD, A. P. M. 1962. The osmoregulation of the Crustacea. *Biol. Rev.*, **37**, 257–307.

105. LOCKWOOD, A. P. M. 1968. *Aspects of the physiology of crustacea.* Oliver and Boyd, Edinburgh.

106. — and RIEGEL, J. A. 1969. The excretion of magnesium by *Carcinus maenas. J. exp. Biol.*, **51**, 575–589.

107. — and — Unpublished studies.

108. MADDRELL, S. H. P. 1963. Excretion in the blood-sucking bug, *Rhodnius prolixus* Stål. I. The control of diuresis. *J. exp. Biol.*, **40**, 247–256.

109. — 1964a. Excretion in the blood-sucking bug, *Rhodnius prolixus* Stål. II. The normal course of diuresis and the effect of temperature. *J. exp. Biol.*, **41**, 163–176.

110. — 1964b. Excretion in the blood-sucking bug, *Rhodnius prolixus* Stål. III. The control of the release of the diuretic hormone. Ibid, 459–472.

111. — 1966a. Nervous control of the mechanical properties of the abdominal wall at feeding in *Rhodnius. J. exp. Biol.*, **44**, 59–68.

112. — 1966b. The site of release of the diuretic hormone in *Rhodnius*— a new neurohaemal system in insects. *J. exp. Biol.*, **45**, 499–508.

113. — Personal communication.

114. — 1969. Secretion by the Malpighian tubules of *Rhodnius*. The movements of ions and water. *J. exp. Biol.*, **51**, 71–97.

115. — PILCHER, D. E., and GARDNER, B. O. C. 1969. Stimulating effect of 5-hydroxytryptamine (serotonin) on secretion by Malpighian tubules of insects. *Nature, Lond.*, **222**, 784–785.

116. MALACZYŃSKA-SUCHCITZ, Z., and UCIŃSKI, B. 1962. Cythophysiological and cytochemical investigation on the epithelium of the antennal gland of the crayfish *Astacus. Folia Biol.*, **10**, 251–292.

117. MALNIC, G., KLOSE, R. M., and GIEBISCH, G. 1966. Micropuncture study of distal tubular potassium and sodium transport in rat nephron. *Am. J. Physiol.*, **211**, 529–547.

118. MALUF, N. S. R. 1941. Secretion of inulin, xylose and dyes and its bearing on the manner of urine-formation by the kidney of the crayfish. *Biol. Bull. Woods Hole*, **81**, 235–260.

118A. MALVIN, R. L., CAFRONI, E. J., and KUTCHAI, H. 1965. Renal transport of glucose by the aglomerular fish *Lophius americanus. J. cell. comp. Physiol.*, **65**, 381–384.

119. MANN, K. H. 1961. *The leeches.* Pergamon Press, Oxford.

120. MARSH, D. J. 1966. Hypo-osmotic re-absorption due to active salt transport in the perfused collecting ducts of the rat renal medulla. *Nature, Lond.*, **210**, 1179–1180.

121. — 1970. Solute and water flows in thin limbs of Henle's loop in the hamster kidney. *Am. J. Physiol.*, **218**, 824–831.

122. — and SOLOMON, S. 1965. Analysis of electrolyte movement in thin Henle's loops of hamster papilla. *Am. J. Physiol.*, **208**, 1119–1128.

124. MARTIN, A. W. 1957. Recent Advances in knowledge of invertebrate renal function. In *Recent advances in invertebrate physiology.* Univ. Oregon Press.

125. MARTIN, A. W., HARRISON, F. M., *et al.* 1958. The blood volumes of some representative molluscs. *J. exp. Biol.* **35**, 260–279.

126. — STEWART, D. M., and HARRISON, F. M. 1965. Urine formation in the pulmonate land snail, *Achatina fulica*. *J. exp. Biol.*, **42**, 99–124.

128. MASSRY, S. G., COBURN, J. W., *et al.* 1967. Effect of NaCl infusion on urinary Ca^{++} and Mg^{++} during reduction in their filtered loads. *Am. J. Physiol.*, **213**, 1218–1224.

129. MAST, S. O., and FOWLER, C. 1935. Permeability of *Amoeba proteus* to water. *J. cell. comp. Physiol.*, **6**, 151–167.

130. MENEFEE, M. G., and MUELLER, C. B. 1967. Some morphological considerations of transport in the glomerulus. In *Ultrastructure of the kidney*. Academic Press, London and New York.

131. MIYAWAKI, M., and UKESHIMA, A. 1967. On the ultrastructure of the antennal gland epithelium of the crayfish, *Procambarus clarkii*. *Kumamoto J. Sci.*, B, **8**, 59–73.

132. MORGAN, T., and BERLINER, R. W. 1968. Permeability of the loop of Henle, vasa recta, and collecting duct to water, urea, and sodium. *Am. J. Physiol.*, **215**, 108–115.

133. MUNZ, F. W., and McFARLAND, W. N. 1964. Regulatory function of a primitive vertebrate kidney. *Comp. Biochem. Physiol.*, **13**, 381–400.

134. NEUMAN, D. 1960. Osmotische Resistenz und Osmoregulation der Flussdeckelschnecke, *Theodoxus fluviatilis* L. *Zool. Z'bl.*, **79**, 585–605.

135. NOBLE-NESBITT, J. 1970. Water balance in the firebrat, *Thermobia domestica* (Packard). *J. exp. Biol.*, **52**, 193–200.

135A. OGLESBY, L. C. 1969. Inorganic components and metabolism; ionic and osmotic regulation: Annelida, Siponcula, and Echiura. Chapter 9 in *Chemical Zoology*, **4**, M. Florkin and B. T. Scheer, (Eds). Academic Press, London and New York.

136. OKEN, D. E., and SOLOMON, A. K. 1960. Potassium concentration in the proximal tubule of *Necturus* kidney. *J. clin. Invest.*, **39**, 1015.

137. ORLOFF, J., and HANDLER, J. S. 1964. The cellular mode of action of antidiuretic hormone. *Am. J. Med.*, **36**, 686–697.

138. PALADE, G. E. 1961. Blood capillaries of the heart and other organs. *Circulation*, **24**, 368–384.

139. PALM, N.-B. 1952. Storage and excretion of vital dyes in insects. *Ark. Zool.*, **3**, 195–272.

140. — 1953. The elimination of injected vital dyes from the blood in myriapods. *Ark. Zool.*, **6**, 219–246.

141. PANTIN, C. F. A. 1947. The nephridia of *Geonemertes dendyi*. *Q. Jl. microsc. Sci.*, **88**, 15–25.

142. PAPPENHEIMER, J. R. 1953. Passage of molecules through capillary walls. *Physiol. Rev.*, **33**, 387–423.

143. PAPPENHEIMER, J. R., RENKIN, E. M., and BORRERO, L. M. 1951. Filtration, diffusion and molecular sieving through peripheral capillary membranes. *Am. J. Physiol.*, **167**, 13–46.

144. PHILLIPS, J. E. 1964. Rectal absorption in the desert locust, *Schistocerca gregaria* Forskal. I–III. *J. exp. Biol.*, **41**, 15–80.

145. — 1969. Osmotic regulation and rectal absorption in the blowfly, *Calliphora erythrocephala. Can. J. Zool.*, **47**, 851–863.

146. — and DOCKRILL, A. A. 1968. Molecular sieving of hydrophilic molecules by the rectal intima of the desert locust (*Schistocerca gregaria*). *J. exp. Biol.*, **48**, 521–532.

146A. PHILLIPS, M. R. Personal communication.

147. PICKEN, L. E. R. 1936. The mechanism of urine formation in invertebrates. I. The excretion mechanism in certain Arthropoda. *J. exp. Biol.*, **13**, 309–328.

148. — 1937. The mechanism of urine formation in invertebrates. II. The excretory mechanism in certain Mollusca. *J. exp. Biol.*, **14**, 20–34.

149. PILCHER, D. E. M. 1970. Hormonal control of the Malipighian tubules of the stick insect, *Carausius morosus. J. exp. Biol.*, **52**, 653–665.

150. PITTS, R. F. 1938. Excretion of phenol red by the chicken. *J. cell. comp. Physiol.*, **11**, 99–115.

150A. PONTIN, R. M. 1964. A comparative account of the protonephridia of *Asplanchna* (Rotifera) with special reference to the flame bulbs. *Proc. Zool. Soc. Lond.*, **142**, 511–525.

151. POTTS, W. T. W. 1954. The rate of urine formation in *Anodonta cygnea. J. exp. Biol.*, **31**, 614–617.

152. — 1965. Ammonia excretion in *Octopus dolfleini. Comp. Biochem. Physiol.*, **14**, 339–355.

153. — 1967. Excretion in the molluscs. *Biol. Rev.*, **42**, 1–41.

154. — 1968. Osmotic and ionic regulation. *A. Rev. Physiol.*, **30**, 73–104.

155. — and TODD, M. E. 1965. Kidney function in the octopus. *Comp. Biochem. Physiol.*, **16**, 479–489.

156. POULSON, T. L. 1965. Countercurrent multipliers in avian kidneys. *Science.*, **148**, 389–391.

157. PROSSER, C. L., and BROWN, F. A., Jnr. 1961. *Comparative animal physiology*. Saunders, New York.

158. RALL, D. P., and BURGER, J. W. 1967. Some aspects of hepatic and renal excretion in *Myxine. Am. J. Physiol.*, **212**, 354–356.

159. RAMSAY, J. A. 1949a. The osmotic relations of the earthworm. *J. exp. Biol.*, **26**, 46–56.

160. — 1949b. The site of formation of hypotonic urine in the nephridium of *Lumbricus*. Ibid, 65–75.

161. — 1952. The excretion of sodium and potassium by the Malpighian tubules of *Rhodnius. J. exp. Biol.*, **29**, 110–126.

162. — 1953. Active transport of potassium by the Malpighian tubules of insects. *J. exp. Biol.*, **30**, 358–369.

163. RAMSAY, J. A., 1954. Active transport of water by the Malpighian tubules of the stick insect, *Dixippus morosus* (Orthoptera, Phasmidae). *J. exp. Biol.*, **31**, 104–113.

164. — 1955a. The excretory system of the stick insect, *Dixippus morosus* (Orthoptera, Phasmidae). *J. exp. Biol.*, **32**, 183–199.

165. — 1955b. The excretion of sodium, potassium and water by the Malpighian tubules of the stick insect, *Dixippus morosus* (Orthoptera, Phasmidae). Ibid, 200–216.

166. — 1956. Excretion by the Malpighian tubules of the stick insect, *Dixippus morosus* (Orthoptera, Phasmidae): calcium, magnesium, chloride, phosphate and hydrogen ions. *J. exp. Biol.*, **33**, 697–708.

167. — 1958. Excretion by the Malpighian tubules of the stick insect, *Dixippus morosus* (Orthoptera, Phasmidae): amino acids, sugars and urea. *J. exp. Biol.*, **35**, 871–891.

168. — 1964. The rectal complex of the mealworm *Tenebrio molitor*, L. (Coleoptera, Tenebrionidae). *Phil. Trans. R. Soc. Lond.*, B, **248**, 279–314.

169. — and RIEGEL, J. A. 1961. Inulin excretion by Malpighian tubules. *Nature, Lond.*, **191**, 1115.

170. RICHARDS, A. N., and PLANT, O. H., Quoted in ref. 171.

171. — 1939. Processes of urine formation. *Proc. R. Soc., Lond.*, B, **126**, 398–432.

172. RIEGEL, J. A. 1961. The influence of water-loading and low temperature on certain functional aspects of the crayfish antennal gland. *J. exp. Biol.*, **38**, 291–299.

173. — 1963. Micropuncture studies of chloride concentration and osmotic pressure in the crayfish antennal gland. *J. exp. Biol.*, **40**, 487–492.

174. — 1965. Micropuncture studies of the concentrations of sodium, potassium and inulin in the crayfish antennal gland. *J. exp. Biol.*, **42**, 379–384.

175. — 1966a. Micropuncture studies of formed-body secretion by the excretory organs of the crayfish, frog and stick insect. *J. exp. Biol*, **44**, 379–385.

176. — 1966b. Analysis of formed bodies in urine removed from the crayfish antennal gland by micropuncture. Ibid, 387–395.

177. — 1968. Analysis of the distribution of sodium, potassium and osmotic pressure in the urine of crayfishes. *J. exp. Biol.*, **48**, 587–596.

179. — 1970a. *In vitro* studies of fluid and ion movements due to swelling of formed bodies. *Comp. Biochem. Physiol.*, **35**, 843–856.

180. — 1970b. A new model of transepithelial fluid movement with detailed application to fluid movement in the crayfish antennal gland. *Comp. Biochem. Physiol.*, **36**, 403–410.

180A. — 1971. Excretion, Arthropoda. In *Chemical Zoology*, **6**, M. Florkin and B. T. Scheer (Eds). Academic Press, London and New York.

181. RIEGEL, J. A. Unpublished observations.

182. — and KIRSCHNER, L. B. 1960. The excretion of inulin and glucose by the crayfish antennal gland. *Biol. Bull. Woods Hole*, **118**, 296–307.

183. — and LOCKWOOD, A. P. M. 1961. The role of the antennal gland in the osmotic and ionic regulation of *Carcinus maenas*. *J. exp. Biol.*, **38**, 491–499.

184. ROBERTSON, J. D. 1953. Further studies on ionic regulation in marine invertebrates. *J. exp. Biol.*, **30**, 277–296.

185. DE ROUFFIGNAC, C., and MOREL, F. 1969. Micropuncture study of water, electrolytes, and urea movements along the loops of Henle in *Psammomys*. *J. clin. Invest.*, **48**, 474–486.

186. SCHATZMANN, H. J., WINDHAGER, E. E., and SOLOMON, A. K. 1958. Single proximal tubules of the *Necturus* kidney. II. Effect of DNP and ouabain on water reabsorption. *Am. J. Physiol.*, **195**, 570–574.

187. SCHMIDT-NIELSEN, B., and DAVIS, L. E. 1968. Fluid transport and tubular intercellular spaces in reptilian kidneys. *Science*, **159**, 1105–1108.

188. See reference 191a.

189. SCHMIDT-NIELSEN, B., and LAWS, D. 1963. Invertebrate mechanisms for diluting and concentrating the urine. *A. Rev. Physiol.*, **25**, 631–658.

190. — and O'DELL, R. 1961. Structure and concentrating mechanism in the mammalian kidney. *Am. J. Physiol.*, **200**, 1119–1124.

191. — and SCHRAUGER, C. R. 1963. *Amoeba proteus:* Studying the contractile vacuole by micropuncture. *Science*, **139**, 606–607.

191A. — GERTZ, K. H., and DAVIS, L. E. 1968. Excretion and ultrastructure of the antennal gland of the fiddler crab *Uca mordax*. *J. Morph.*, **125**, 473–495.

192. SCHNEIDER, L. 1960. Electronenmikroskopische Untersuchungen über das Nephridialsystem von Paramecium. *J. Protozool.*, **7**, 75–101.

193. SILVERMAN, M., AGANON, M. A., and CHINARD, F. P. 1970a. D-glucose interactions with renal cell tubular surfaces. *Am. J. Physiol.*, **218**, 735–742.

194. — — and — 1970b. Specificity of monasaccharide transport in dog kidney. Ibid, 743–750.

195. SKADHAUGE, E., and SCHMIDT-NIELSEN, B. 1967. Renal medullary electrolyte and urea gradient in chickens and turkeys. *Am. J. Physiol.*, **212**, 1313–1318.

196. SKELDING, J. M. 1972. Renal function in *Achatina achatina* (L.) and *Helix pomatia* (L.). Doctoral thesis, Univ. of London.

198. SLOTKOFF, L. M., and LILIENFIELD, L. S. 1967. Extravascular renal albumen. *Am. J. Physiol.*, **212**, 400–406.

199. SMITH, H. W. 1951. *The kidney*. Oxford Univ. Press.

200. SMITH, L. S. 1962. Some aspects of peripheral circulation in *Octopus dolfleini*. Ph.D. Thesis, University of Washington.

201. SOLOMON, A. K. 1960. Red cell membrane structure and ion transport. *J. gen. Physiol.*, **43**, (Suppl.), 1–15.

202. SPITZER, A., and WINDHAGER, E. E. 1970. Effect of peritubular oncotic pressure changes on proximal tubular fluid reabsorption. *Am. J. Physiol.*, **218**, 1188–1193.

203. STAVERMAN, A. J. 1951. The theory of the measurement of osmotic pressure. *Receuil des Travaux Chimiques des Pays-Bas*, **70**, 344–352.

204. STOBBART, R. H., and Shaw, J. 1964. Salt and water balance: excretion. In *The physiology of insecta*, **3**. Academic Press, London and New York.

205. STORER, T. I., and USINGER, R. L. 1957. *General zoology*, 3rd. edn. McGraw-Hill, London and New York.

206. TAKEUCHI, T., IIDAKA, K., *et al.* 1961. Renal lymphatics, morphologic approach. *Acta Pathol. Japon.* **11**, 270.

207. THOENES, W. 1968. Neue Befunde zur Beschaffenheit des basalen Labyrinthes im Nierentubulus. *Z. Zellforsch (Histochemie)*, **86**, 351–363.

208. THURAU, K., and HENNE, G. 1963. Dynamik des Harnstromes in der Henleschen Schleife der Goldhamsterniere. *Arch. ges. Physiol.*, **278**, 45–46.

209. — VALTIN, H., and SCHNERMANN, J. 1968. Kidney. *A. Rev. Physiol.*, **30**, 442–524.

209A. — WILDE, W. S., HENNE, G., SCHNERMANN, J., and PRCHAL, K. Quoted in 46A.

210. TODD, M. E. 1964. Osmotic balance in *Hydrobia ulvae* and *Potamopyrgus jenkinsi* (Gastropoda, Hydrobeidae). *J. exp. Biol.*, **41**, 665–677.

211. TORELLI, G., MILLA, E., *et al.* 1966. Energy requirement for sodium reabsorption in the *in vivo* rabbit kidney. *Am. J. Physiol.*, **211**, 576–580.

212. TORMEY, J. McD., and DIAMOND, J. M. 1967. The ultrastructural route of fluid transport in rabbit gall bladder. *J. gen. Physiol.*, **50**, 2131–2060.

213. TYSON, G. E. 1968. The fine structure of the maxillary gland of the brine shrimp, *Artemia salina:* The end-sac. *Z. Zellforsch.*, **86**, 129–138.

214. — 1969a. The fine structure of the maxillary gland of the brine shrimp, *Artemia salina:* The efferent duct. *Z. Zellforsch.*, **93**, 151–163.

215. — 1969b. Intercoil connections of the kidney of the brine shrimp, *Artemia salina. Z. Zellforsch.*, **100**, 54–59.

216. —. Personal communication.

217. ULLRICH, K. J., and MARSH, D. J. 1963. Kidney, water and electrolyte metabolism. *A. Rev. Physiol.*, **25**, 91–142.

218. UNGER, H. 1965. Der Einfluss der Neurohormone C und D auf die Farbstoffabsorptionsfahigkeit der Malpighischen Gefasse (und des Darmes) der Stabheusschrecke *Carausius morosus* (Br.) *in vitro. Zool. Jb. Physiol.*, **71**, 710–717.

219. VORWOHL, G. 1961. Zur Funktion der Excretionsorgane von *Helix pomatia* L. und *Archachatina ventricosa* Gould. *Z. vergl. Physiol.*, **45**, 12–49.

220. WALKER, A. M., BOTT, P. A., *et al.* 1941. The collection and analysis of fluid from single nephrons of the mammalian kidney. *Am. J. Physiol.*, **134**, 580–595.

221. — and OLIVER, J. 1941. Methods for the collection of fluid from single glomeruli and tubules of the mammalian kidney. *Am. J. Physiol.*, **134**, 562–571.

222. WALL, B. J. 1965. Regulation of water metabolism by the Malpighian tubules and rectum in the cockroach *Periplaneta americana* L. *Zool. Jb. Physiol.*, **71**, 702–709.

223. — and OSCHMAN, J. L. 1970. Water and solute uptake by rectal pads of *Periplaneta americana. Am. J. Physiol.*, **218**, 1208–1215.

224. — and RALPH, C. L. 1964. Evidence for hormonal regulation of Malpighian tubule excretion in the insect, *Periplaneta americana* L. *Gen. Comp. Endocrin.*, **4**, 452–456.

225. WALLENIUS, G. 1954. Renal clearance of dextran as a measure of glomerular permeability. *Acta Soc. med. Upsal.* **59**, Suppl. 4.

226. WARNER, F. D. 1969. The fine structure of the protonephridium in the rotifer *Asplanchna. J. Ultrastruct. Res.*, **29**, 499–524.

227. WEARN, J. T., and RICHARDS, A. N. 1924. Observations on the composition of glomerular urine, with particular reference to the problem of reabsorption in the renal tubules. *Am. J. Physiol.*, **71**, 209–227.

228. WHITTEMBURY, G. 1960. Ion and water transport in the proximal tubules of the kidney of *Necturus maculosus. J. gen. Physiol.*, **43**, (Suppl.), 43–56.

229. WHITTEMBURY, G., OKEN, D. E., WINDHAGER, E. E. *et al.* 1959. Single proximal tubules of *Necturus* kidney. IV. Dependence of H_2O movements on osmotic gradients. *Am. J. Physiol.*, **197**, 1121–1127.

230. WIGGLESWORTH, V. B. 1931. The physiology of excretion in a blood-sucking insect, *Rhodnius prolixus* (Hemiptera, Reduviidae). I–III. *J. exp. Biol.*, **8**, 411–451.

231. WIGGLESWORTH, V. B. 1932. On the function of the so-called 'rectal glands' of insects. *Q. Jl. microsc. Sci.*, **75**, 131–150.

232. WIGGLESWORTH, V. B. 1934. *Insect physiology*. Methuen, London.

233. WINDHAGER, E. E. 1964. Electrophysiological study of the renal papilla of golden hamsters. *Am. J. Physiol.*, **206**, 694–700.

234. — 1968. *Micropuncture techniques and nephron function*. Butterworths, London.

235. WINDHAGER, E. E. 1969. Kidney, water and electrolytes. *A. Rev. Physiol.*, **31**, 117–172.

236. — and GIEBISCH, G. 1961. Micropuncture study of renal tubular transfer of sodium chloride in the rat. *Am. J. Physiol.*, **200**, 581–590.

237. — WHITTEMBURY, G., *et al.* 1959. Single proximal tubules of the *Necturus* kidney. III. Dependence of H_2O movement on NaCl concentration. *Am. J. Physiol.*, **197**, 313–318.

238. WIRZ, H. HARGITAY, B., and KUHN, W. 1951. Lokalisation des Konzentrierungsprozesses in der Niere durch direkte Kryoskopie. *Helv. physiol. pharmac. Acta*, **9**, 196–207.

Index

N.B. Numbers in bold refer to definitions

Abbreviations: T. = table, F. = figure, ff. = following page(s).